Please Stay

Please Stay

A BRAIN BLEED, A LIFE IN THE
BALANCE, A LOVE STORY

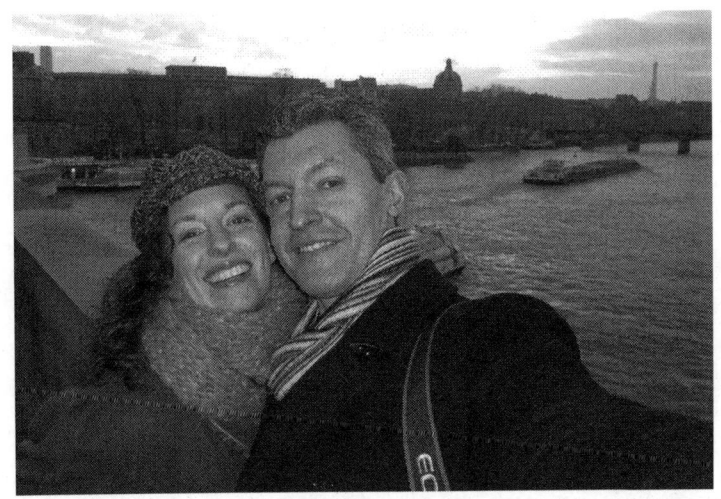

Greg Payan

© 2017 Greg Payan
All rights reserved.

ISBN-13: 9781540493736
ISBN-10: 1540493733
Library of Congress Control Number: 2016919507
CreateSpace Independent Publishing Platform
North Charleston, South Carolina

Acknowledgments

FIRST AND FOREMOST, THIS BOOK would not have been possible if not for Dr. David Chalif, chief of neurosurgery at Long Island Jewish Medical Center in Manhasset, New York (today known as Northwell Health). His skill and steady hand not only saved Holly's life but also gave her back the life she lived—with no deficits and against all odds. There are no appropriate words of gratitude for someone who saves the life of one's partner, nor will there ever be. *Thank you* will have to do.

I am so grateful to Nicole Salant of the neuro unit, who answered every question with kindness and always had a hug for us on follow-up visits. To the entire neurological staff at Long Island Jewish and the neuro ICU nurses under the guidance of Laura Iacono: Thank you so much for the phenomenal care and compassion you showed to Holly and to our family and for the grace you show daily as you deal with some of medicine's most difficult cases. Every day in the ICU, you provided the best of care to Holly and emotional sustenance to my family and me.

To Sharley, my sister-in-law who's more like my sister: You were strong when I was weak and calm when I was anxious. You made it clear where Holly gets her strength. There is nobody stronger than Frank and Susan Hillgardner's girls.

To my parents, Michel and Diana: As you have for my entire life, you went above and beyond the call of duty. During this crisis, you spent countless hours in the ICU and took care of me in those first weeks when I stayed with you to be close to the hospital. I am also eternally grateful for the way you nursed Holly back to health after her many subsequent surgeries so that I could spend necessary time at work. You both are truly the best.

To my brothers, Mike and Chris: thank you for your love, support, and prayers. To Charlie, Brian, Kieran, Alex, and Elvis—friends from back in the day: thank you for your words of encouragement and daily prayers, which gave me a spiritual lift I often could not give myself. To Tommy, Ann, Em, and Katie: thank you for being there through this ordeal and throughout my life.

To the neuro staff at New York University Langone Medical Center, especially Dr. Dimitris G. Placantonakis, who finally got Holly's shunt right after the first three needed to be replaced through no fault of any doctor: we are so grateful for the care we received, as complications arose in the months after Holly's ICU stay and rehab and were resolved at a different hospital.

To Holly's New York "brainsitters" Karen, Christy, Cynthia, and Demy, you were wonderful in keeping Holly company at the hospital and then spending countless hours with her at home when I needed to go to work. Christy gets bonus points for being my first sounding board/editor on one of the early drafts of this book. Along with being a fabulous scholar, friend, and mom, you provided invaluable early feedback. I also thank Chatman Neely for looking over my first (and likely pretty awful) draft of this book and emphasizing the importance of making my voice more prominent.

To Keely Patridge, our long-distance brainsitter: You flew halfway across the country, slept on our couch for a week, and kept a smile on your face the whole time while helping me take care of Holly. The laughter and positivity you provided that first week out of rehab lasted long after you returned home. I will forever cherish you for doing that.

To Erin Adwell Teague, who lovingly organized a fundraiser for Holly in her old hometown just as bills were starting to mount.

To all of our many friends and family not mentioned here by name who reached out via texts, e-mails, and phone calls: Your notes were like oxygen to me on my darkest days. I feel that those communications, many of which are included in this book, are what makes this story special.

To my employer, the Associated Press, and my work colleagues: thank you for being so accommodating of my need to spend as much time as possible at hospitals and rehab centers throughout Holly's many surgeries and recoveries.

To Catherine Keller: thank you for unknowingly providing the title for this book in a letter to Holly and for the counsel and friendship that have fueled Holly throughout her academic career.

Lastly, I thank you, Holly. You brighten my every day as we walk through this world together.

> *Someday, the light will shine like a sun through my skin*
> *and they will say,*
> *What have you done with your life? And*
> *though there are many moments*
> *I think I will remember, in the end, I will be proudest to say,*
> *I was one of us.*
>
> —Brian Andreas

For the caregivers who did not have my outcome:
I am humbled by your strength.
I am amazed at your dedication.
I am in awe at how you move forward
in the face of what has been thrust upon you.

Prologue

"This is the best time I ever had."

She didn't mean it literally. She used the line too often. Not so often that it lost meaning but often enough—a few times a year in your presence if you were lucky. When you heard it, you knew it wasn't *the* best time she'd ever had, but you sure as hell knew life at that moment was pretty close to perfect.

She might say it while eating churros sold out of the back of a truck on the Pacific coast of Mexico. Or maybe while having a martini freshly shaken by a waitress at a roadside BBQ joint in Bali. Or maybe while doing something closer to home, such as enjoying lamb biryani takeout at night on the balcony of her tiny Manhattan studio on a warm summer evening. "This is the best time I ever had." Every time I heard her say it, it was validation—I was a part of the life she wanted to be living. It also meant I was part of the life *I* wanted to be living too, as a partner in a committed relationship with someone who I thought was the greatest woman in the world.

In 2014, I was forty-two years old and living in a one-bedroom apartment in Queens, New York. I drove a beat-up 1998 Honda that was usually clean only when it rained, but who cared? I was in love with a fabulous woman whom I had adored for more than a decade—my fiancée, Holly. We both had jobs we loved. I worked in the photo sales and licensing department at the Associated Press in New York, and she was a professor of religious studies at Bethany College in West Virginia. We were fully committed and yet independent. We spent school semesters apart, but we were together as much as possible on weekends and school breaks. In many ways, we lived an enchanted life—supporting each other from near and far and truly believing we were our best selves because of each other. After ten years with her, my heart would still race when she bounced into baggage claim as I waited to pick her up after her latest flight. I was living a schoolboy crush in the real world as an adult but in a wonderful, equal partnership.

Holly was a vibrant thirty-nine-year-old woman—happy, healthy, and never having endured any serious illness or surgery to that point in her life. She was a yoga teacher who, before getting her PhD, had spent a decade teaching high school English in Texas and in the South Bronx, New York. Holly loved the ocean, her friends, teaching, collecting passport stamps from around the world, and surfing small waves, which she did with an ear-to-ear smile across her face.

If you're lucky, one person like Holly might come into your life—someone who makes everything you do with them just a bit better than if you did it with anyone else. She forced me to think and made me care about things I'd never thought I'd care about. Holly made me live my life deeper than I ever thought possible, and she was everything to me.

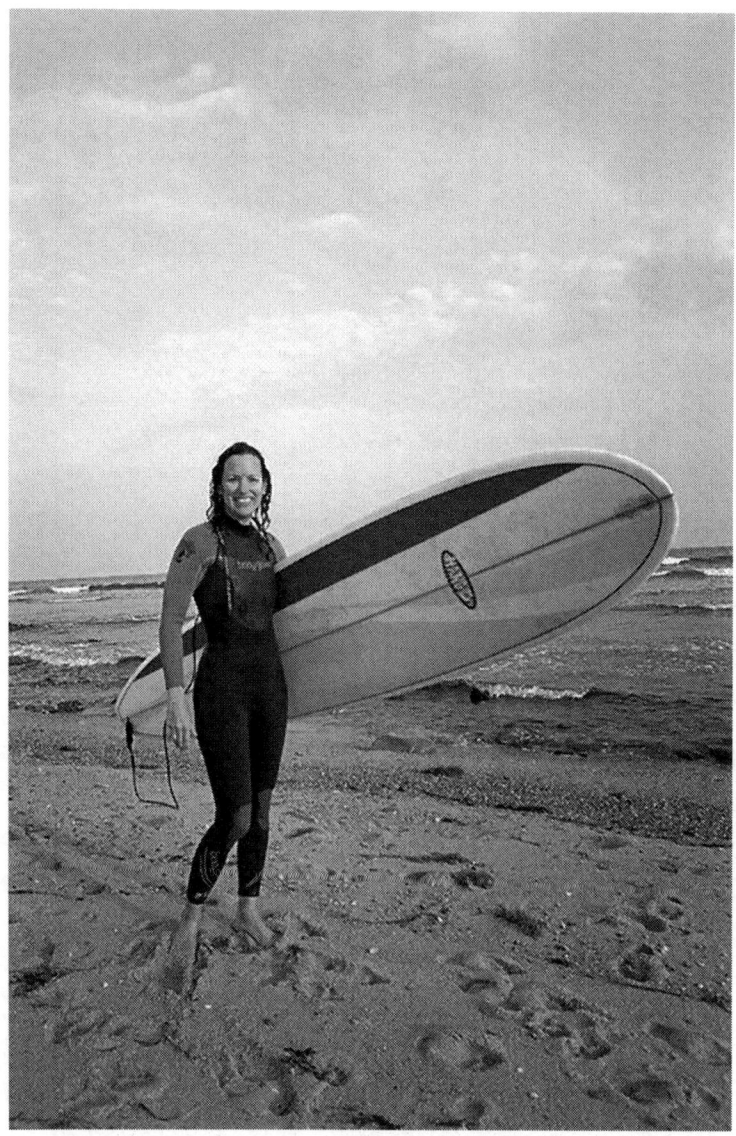

Holly at Ditch Plains in Montauk, New York, July 2012.

On the day after Easter in April 2014, my world shattered. At 5:30 a.m., Holly awoke with a ruptured aneurysm in her brain. She was unable to move and barely able to speak. It is not hyperbole to say she almost did not survive.

She suffered heart and lung failure as she ceased breathing on her own as blood leaked from the rupture into her skull. In the days and weeks that followed, I also was informed that rare is the instance where a person fully recovers from an aneurysm rupture, and often the recovery can take years. I thought Holly might make it through this if she was lucky, but the life we were living was soon to be a distant memory for all intents and purposes.

A brain aneurysm is a weak spot on the wall of an artery in the brain. Over time, as the artery wall gradually becomes thinner from dilation, blood flow causes the weakened wall to balloon outward. This pressure may cause the aneurysm to rupture; if this happens, blood will hemorrhage into the space around the brain. Brain hemorrhages caused by a ruptured aneurysm often occur with little or no warning, and they nearly always require lifesaving intervention be administered as soon as possible if someone hopes to survive.

According to the Brain Aneurysm Foundation, 15 percent of people in whom an aneurysm ruptures die before they receive medical care, and another 25 percent die within twenty-four hours of arriving at a hospital. The possibility of death depends on the severity of the bleed, the location of the aneurysm, and how quickly the person is treated. If someone is lucky enough to survive the initial bleed, a myriad of complications can cause death in the weeks of intensive care that follow. Of those who live, about 66 percent suffer some permanent neurological deficit, according to the foundation. Despite the fact that aneurysms are seemingly an under-the-radar killer, they cause almost five hundred thousand deaths worldwide each year. Half of the victims are younger than fifty.

Holly's aneurysm ruptured without warning. We'd never known she had one. She barely survived that day and spent twenty-four days in the intensive care unit, fighting for her life during much of that time. During those critical weeks, I solicited letters from friends and family, and I read many of these notes to Holly during her various states of lucidity and consciousness. They were beautiful and heartbreaking; they illustrated the impact she'd had as a schoolteacher, a professor, a scholar, and a friend. She had influenced countless lives. This book includes many of those letters, because they became a part of the journey—a journey that began with Holly near death and facing almost certain disability if she survived. Alongside these letters is my real-time narrative of this ordeal—the panic, the confusion, the waiting, the anxiety, and the tears. Also included are dozens of text messages I exchanged with Sharley, Holly's sister, who spent countless hours at the hospital with me during the crisis.

At some point of every day of Holly's ICU stay, I sent an e-mail to family and friends, updating them on Holly's condition. My notes were a bit maudlin. In retrospect, they seem out of character for me. But they clearly reflect my mood and thinking at the time—emotionally on edge, sleep-deprived, constantly sick with worry, and desperate for Holly to somehow live through this and get well.

Holly survived. She made it through a ruptured aneurysm and all the complications that followed. Her official medical diagnosis was a grade IV subarachnoid hemorrhage, the result of a ruptured aneurysm on her basilar artery. I knew her recovery was miraculous, but a conversation months later best illustrated how rare it actually was.

While we were in the emergency room at New York University Langone Medical Center for treatment of one of Holly's many complications in the months after her initial bleed, a neurosurgeon interviewed us about Holly's medical history. When informed Holly had endured a grade IV brain hemorrhage, he refused to believe it. He began educating us on how the grading system works, but I interrupted him, saying we knew how it worked. I told him that yes, Holly had survived a grade IV brain hemorrhage just five months prior.

His eyes widened as he looked at Holly again. "You don't see people present like she does after a grade IV hemorrhage," he said. "You should consider yourself extremely lucky."

I said we had been told many times that she was doing well, and we were incredibly grateful.

He persisted, shaking his head. "You don't understand. We have a sad saying here. We say that eighty percent of people who have a grade IV brain hemorrhage die. And of those that live, eighty percent *wish* they had died."

Part 1
A Crisis Unfolding

DAY 1 — BRAIN BLEED
April 21, 2014

In the early morning hours on Monday, April 21, 2014, Holly was finishing up a trip to New York City for the weekend, and I was getting ready to take her to the airport for her flight to West Virginia to teach her midday class. I always got up first when she had flights home, letting her enjoy as much sleep as possible. I would make her coffee and breakfast, so she could roll out of bed and into our car without having to waste precious sleep time getting ready. While brushing my teeth that morning, I heard her crying in our bedroom, so I went to check on her.

I had no way of understanding the gravity of the situation in that moment, even though she was unable to move. I was more confused than scared, trying to understand why someone would be incapacitated by a headache, and I thought only of my mother, who had struggled with migraines throughout my youth. They often left my mother bedridden, though never like this. I wondered if Holly could be having a migraine, although she'd never had one before. I would learn later that Holly had harbored a brain aneurysm, and it had burst without warning as she slept.

5:40 a.m.
My text to Sharley, Holly's sister:
Are you awake?
Holly woke up really sick and needs to talk to you.

The e-mail I sent to my work colleagues:
From: Payan, Gregory
Sent: Monday, April 21, 2014, 5:44 a.m.
Subject: Greg Monday

All:
Holly woke up really sick and is going to miss her flight. I am on standby to take her to the doctor. Will be on e-mail periodically through morn and need to take a personal day.
Greg

5:55 a.m.
Sharley's text to me:
Hold on. I'm waking her up. (This is Dave)

Sharley called me after her husband woke her, but almost immediately after I answered the phone, Holly began to convulse. I hung up on Shar and called 911. Holly's eyes rolled back in her head, and she moaned with a low, guttural sound. She was unresponsive for about twenty seconds. I held her upright as she continued to moan, and in a loud whisper, I said into her ear, "No! No! No! Don't you dare fucking die on me, Holly. I don't know what's going on, but you're going to get through this, and we're going to live a long life together. I know you hear me. Don't you die."

I tried to calm down, but I was scared she would stop breathing in my arms and go totally limp at any moment. I truly thought her life might end right there. Then, slowly, she became somewhat responsive again. A nontechnical way to describe things was that her brain had short-circuited for a minute or two.

Five minutes after I called 911, an ambulance arrived, and Holly became a bit more aware of her surroundings, although she was in seemingly worse pain. The emergency medical technicians who took us to the hospital a mile away appeared to be unconcerned, as if they thought she was only experiencing a bad headache. They even reminded me to bring her shoes, so she would not be barefoot when she walked out of the ER later that day. Holly was in only her pajamas—a black tank top and a pair of my oversized gray sweatpants, rolled at the waist so they would not fall off.

Holly's vital signs were stable in the ambulance. She had a normal blood-pressure reading and stable heart rate, although she was in terrible pain. When we arrived at the hospital, nobody seemed hurried, which was probably due to the EMTs' apparent apathy. I was ready to crawl out of my skin. I held Holly's hand as she lay on a gurney in the emergency room, watching the second hand on the clock as I waited for a doctor to come over. I called Shar, Holly's sister, who worked as an EMT herself, and told her how critical I thought the situation was. She told me to find the resident on duty and beg for a CT scan.

I walked over to the resident. "Good morning," I said softly. "I know there are many sick people in here now and relatives who feel their loved one isn't being treated fast enough, but my fiancée is really sick. Her vitals are stable, and she's conscious, but she has a terrible headache, can't move because of the pain, and was convulsing half an hour ago. Her sister is an EMT and feels she desperately needs a CT scan. Can you please get this test done? She's very sick, and I think she's having a brain bleed or something like that." I was as respectful as I could be, and it worked. He stopped what he was doing and immediately took her to another room.

I waited. After about fifteen minutes, the resident returned with a look of grave concern. He told me Holly was having a brain hemorrhage, and she would be transferred by ambulance to a facility ten miles away for emergency surgery. I was to follow in a cab. The resident told me to get her family and "anyone important in her life" to the other hospital as quickly as possible.

I had just a few moments to try to explain to Holly what was happening. I wanted to project confidence in spite of the gravity of the situation, even though she was not processing much because of the pain. She was curled up in the fetal position on a gurney.

"It hurts so bad," she said.

"I know it hurts, but they are going to take you to another hospital and fix everything. They are getting the ambulance now. I can't ride with you, but I'll be right behind you in a cab," I whispered, almost up against her face so she could feel my breath close to her.

"Honey, it hurts so bad," she said again.

I kissed her cheek.

"Owww," she moaned, barely loudly enough for me to hear her.

"I love you. You're gonna be OK. I promise. We got this," I said.

Two men in scrubs came by. "I'm sorry, but we have to go right now."

I squeezed her hand and whispered in her ear, "I love you." I kissed her more softly this time.

They wheeled her away. I took a huge, deep breath, wondering if this was the end. It was all so abrupt. An hour earlier, I'd been brushing my teeth after making Holly a cup of coffee. Now I may have just seen her alive for the last time. "What the hell is happening?" I thought, as the administrative person behind the desk called a cab to take me to the next hospital half an hour away.

After an awkward ride that seemed to take an eternity in rush hour traffic to Long Island where my cab driver played the role of therapist, I arrived at the second hospital. I identified myself to the receptionist. She gave me a horrified look. "Hold on," she said. For a few seconds, I thought I was too late.

She summoned a social worker, who advised me that Holly's condition had deteriorated significantly in the ambulance ride over; she had stopped breathing en route and had to be intubated. The social worker asked if I wanted to speak to a priest.

I said no, but I felt an incredible urge to talk with someone, so I gratefully accepted the social worker's company. She sat with me, looked at photos on my phone, and listened as I told her all the special things about Holly that made me love her. Subconsciously, I may have been practicing for the eulogy I thought I might be giving soon.

Holly and I had met on a beach in Zihuatanejo, Mexico, in the summer of 2004. I had just separated from my wife, and Holly had just broken off an engagement. We were both traveling alone—doing some soul-searching and hoping for a bit of healing. On a hot, lazy afternoon, we wound up on Playa La Ropa under separate beach umbrellas. I noticed her from a distance. I saw, quite simply, a pretty girl in a bikini reading a book. Hoping she was another single traveler, I wandered over and delivered what Holly insists was the best pickup line someone could offer an English teacher: "What are you reading?"

Dinner followed that evening, along with a late-night swim. It was wonderful, but our time together was brief. The following day, I had to board a plane. We exchanged e-mail addresses and a goodbye kiss, although we both thought it was possible we would never see each other again. Holly lived in Texas, and I lived in New York. Even if I never saw her again, I thought, at least I'd have this photo, taken by our waiter at dinner that night. It pictures two happy travelers at the end of a nice meal, red-faced from the Mexican sun, a few glasses of wine, and the ninety-degree temperature and high humidity that lingered long into the evening.

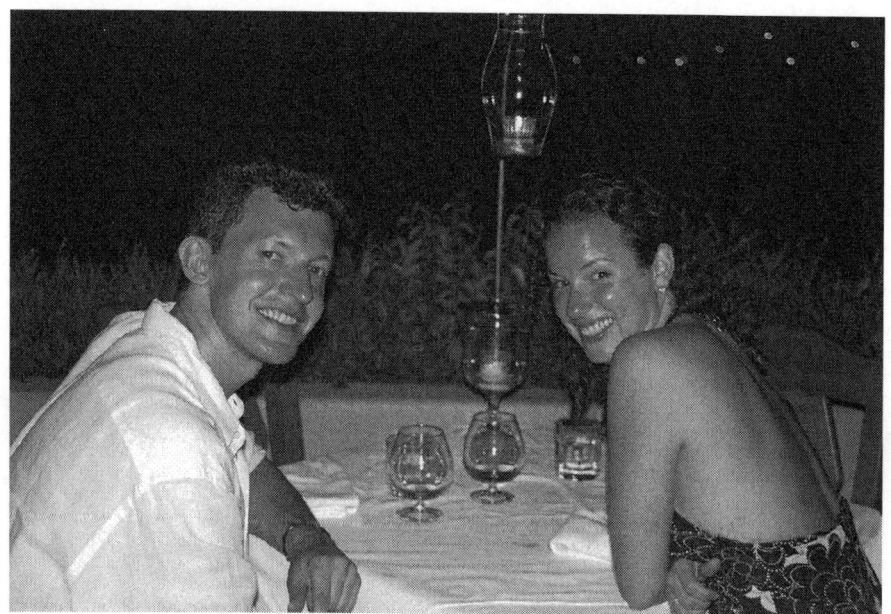

Our first date in Zihuatanejo, Mexico, in June 2004.

After flying home and returning to the office the following day, I was pleasantly surprised to see the following e-mail arrive in my mailbox after lunch:

From:	Holly
Sent:	Wednesday, June 16, 2004, 1:05 p.m.
To:	Greg
Subject:	Vida sans Greg en Zihua

Greg

Here's a quick list of what I have done since you left:

1. I have dreamily lay on the beach.
2. I have gotten sentimental about yellow Japanese sandals that don't fit.
3. I have found the bakery you mentioned and the Internet café.
4. I have contracted a very strange rash on my hand (which I am sure has nothing to do with you!).
5. I have generally not been myself.

Your list?
Holly

Her short, flirty correspondence was validation that she had enjoyed my company as much as I had hers. We'd purchased the sandals Holly referred to the morning of my flight. The tide had stolen hers during our swim the night before. We had limited options at a tiny beachside store, so I bought a pair sized for children's feet, so she would not be barefoot.

In the following weeks, we exchanged e-mails and agreed we really did want to see each other again. I remember telling my mother about Holly the week I returned from Mexico: "We only spent a day together, but I really think she's gonna be around in my life for a long time."

Our second meeting was in Vermont six weeks later. I was to be her date for her sister's wedding. Over the coming months, we saw each other as much as possible, alternating visits. I flew to Texas to see her, she flew to New York to see me, and we threw a New Year's trip to Barcelona into the mix as well.

However improbable it may have seemed at the start, a relationship developed. A year after we met in Mexico, Holly got a job teaching English in the South Bronx and moved to New York. For a time, we were happy together. Yet our relationship eventually turned stormy. Holly and I are two very independent people, and we had trouble wrapping our lives around a partnership. After three years, these issues led us to take a three-week break and then a longer one of about eight months. During these breaks, neither of us was fully able to move on emotionally, although we convinced ourselves many times that we had.

The time apart turned out to be helpful. We gave our relationship another try after we'd both had a bit of therapy, and suddenly our time together was happy and peaceful. The best parts of our relationship remained, and the issues were simply gone. Our lives became intertwined, and we embraced that instead of rebelling against it, as we had previously. In the years that followed, we were living our dreams—we both had jobs we loved and wonderful friends. We enjoyed traveling the world together, near and far, whenever our schedules allowed.

Hell, we didn't even fight anymore. Maybe we engaged in some occasional playful bickering, but fighting? I could not even remember the last time we'd raised our voices to each other. Don't get me wrong; Holly was headstrong, and I could argue, but it was predictable and always had to do with one of two things: The first thing that made her insane was my car's GPS, which Holly sometimes referred to as "the other woman." I have absolutely no sense of direction and am utterly reliant on my GPS to get from point A to point B, regardless of how many times I have traversed the route before. She would often joke that I would follow directions blindly into a lake, a telephone pole, or even oncoming traffic if my GPS directed me to. The second thing that could get Holly going was luggage. You see, Holly believed that all good travelers should be able to go anywhere in the world with just carry-on luggage. For example, she went to India for two months with only a duffel bag. I, however, love to overpack, and I check luggage even for the shortest of trips. I am six feet and three inches tall, and I weigh about 220 pounds. I justify my checked bags by saying to Holly, "I'm a big guy, and my clothes take up a lot of space." Any variation of this statement was all but assured to send her into a fury as I placed my clothing into a large suitcase as we packed for a flight.

There was a time when Holly might get frustrated if I was inarticulate or mixed up words or phrases, but no longer. Now such ridiculousness is greeted with a smile and a gentle exclamation of "word salad," which alerts me that what I've said was quite unintelligible to anyone other than us. Holly will then insist she is the only one who could ever understand me.

Holly and I assumed we would get married someday. Maybe sooner or maybe later. Maybe in Montauk. Or maybe on a beach in India. We were sometimes "boyfriend and girlfriend," other times "partners," and still other times "fiancé and fiancée," but we were not in a hurry to have a wedding. We had been fully committed for many years. We'd even had wills and health-care proxies drawn up in 2012 after Holly had a kidney stone—we'd realized I could have been asked to leave her hospital room at any time. A lawyer friend drew up the paperwork, and I gave Holly a ring to commemorate the signing of our wills and health-care proxies—a ring she called her "rocksy-proxy" ring that she wore on her left ring finger.

On April 21, in the hospital, I was almost certain that if Holly did not die, she would be nothing like the person she'd been the day before. She was in the midst of a severe brain hemorrhage, and I could not wrap my head around what this could mean in the moment, much less the future. The main thing I was hoping was that my phone would not run out of battery power as I sat with the social worker, showing her picture after picture from my phone's camera and from our Facebook pages. Holly was my world. She was a person—the best person—and I needed anyone who administered care to her to want her to live as much as I did, with every ounce of his or her being. I wanted them to know and understand that they had to bring her back. Listening to me patiently, the social worker was an angel, as were so many of Holly's caregivers at the hospital. At the worst time in my life, these strangers comforted me. I was humbled by the empathy they showed me day after day during the journey that followed.

I'd spent about an hour with the social worker when a doctor finally came out and told me Holly was in poor shape. Her aneurysm had ruptured, resulting in a severe brain hemorrhage. He'd put a drain in, and his team would try to stabilize her over the next few hours. The situation was extremely critical. He did not mince words or express fake optimism. Holly may or may not live. He did not know what condition she would be in if she did make it. I thanked him, took a few deep breaths, and went to the neuro ICU waiting room to wait for further updates.

The Hunt and Hess Scale describes the severity of a subarachnoid hemorrhage and is used as a predictor of survival. Even the lowest-grade hemorrhage carries a high risk of death, irrespective of deficits or issues that could plague victims for the rest of their lives. Holly had experienced a Grade IV hemorrhage. Symptoms and survival rates are listed below:

Grade I

- asymptomatic or minimal headache and slight neck stiffness
- 70 percent survival rate

Grade II

- moderate to severe headache
- neck stiffness
- no neurologic deficit except cranial nerve palsy
- 60 percent survival rate

Grade III

- drowsiness / confusion
- mild focal neurologic deficit
- 50 percent survival rate

Grade IV

- stuporous
- moderate to severe hemiparesis (muscle weakness or paralysis)
- possibly early decerebrate rigidity and vegetative disturbances
- 20 percent survival rate

Grade V

- deep coma
- decerebrate rigidity / moribund
- 10 percent survival rate

8:21 a.m.
Shar texted me:
Can I call your parents to come wait with you?

I replied to Shar:
I called. They are coming.

Shar texted me:
OK good. Where are you now?

I replied:
ICU waiting room.

The social worker who had sat with me for the last hour escorted me to the fourth floor of the hospital, where the Neuro ICU was. The waiting room was down the hall. She gave me a hug and left just before I entered the room. I walked into a rather nondescript room with about fifteen or twenty seats, half of them filled. On the wall just when I walked in was a phrase in big white letters: "Believe in Miracles." I took a picture and sent it to Sharley, who by now was on the road en route to New York. A TV mounted to the wall was on, but no sound came from it. The room was windowless and smelled like a hospital, a light scent of disinfectant or bleach, which I guess was understandable. They were trying to save lives, and my comfort was surely not their highest priority. Nobody was in this room unless experiencing the worst of emotions. We all would rather have been anywhere else, as we desperately waited for information on what was happening with a loved one.

My parents had yet to arrive, and I was alone. I looked around at the other people waiting, who seemed to be in various states of breakdowns. Nobody was crying or talking. Just a room for people alone with their thoughts. Maybe—like me—they had gone to bed the night before with everything "normal," only to be shocked by what had transpired in the last few hours. Maybe they had spoken to their loved ones for the last time. Maybe I had too.

Time passed with few answers or updates. Sharley arrived from Massachusetts with her husband, Dave, and young son, Elliot, just before noon. My parents

Please Stay

came, as did a few other family members. I called some of Holly's closest friends to explain what had happened and tried to keep it together. We could tell from the few updates we received that the situation was bad. E-mails of support began to arrive for us.

Rachael e-mailed:
Greg,
I just heard about Holly from Natalie. I am sooo sorry. My thoughts and prayers are with you both. Please let me know if there is ANYTHING I can do at all to help. Anything! I am here for you, Greg.

> **I replied to Rachael:**
> It's bad. Just thoughts and prayers, thanks. Not much info yet. In waiting room. Arterial bleed on brain. Not good.

Charlie e-mailed:
Greg.
Loreen, Kathleen, Kelly, CJ, and I will be praying for Holly over these next few days, praying that everything will go as well as could be expected. You will also be in our prayers because I know this is VERY tough for you as well…hang in there, buddy…God Bless.

> **I replied to Charlie:**
> Thanks. She's a fighter, which is great, but she's real sick.

Kieran e-mailed:
Hey Greg,
   Alex texted me earlier, and I spoke with Brian a few minutes ago about the brain aneurysm that Holly suffered this morning. I will get my three daughters to pray for her…God always listens to little girls. Hang in there,

buddy. I know that these are scary times, but you have to think positive thoughts.

―⸺

This is the report from Holly's first scan at Long Island Jewish Medical Center. In it, the doctor refers to comparing this scan with "the prior study," which is the scan done that morning at Forest Hills, our local hospital, where we went first. In retrospect, I look at this report and am surprised at the size of Holly's aneurysm. It would be regarded as "small" by most neurosurgeons, and even if doctors had discovered the aneurysm before it ruptured, they may have taken a "wait and see" approach regarding her treatment. The other thing that stands out is the reference to "extensive subarachnoid hemorrhage," which usually means dire or tragic consequences.

North Shore University Hospital
Department of Radiology

> Patient: Hillgardner, Holly
> AKA: Hillgardner, Holly
> DOB: 07/01/1974
> AGE: 39Y FEMALE
> Pt. Class: INPATIENT
> Order #: 90006
> Accession#: 28659899

EXAM: BRAIN CT WITHOUT CONTRAST
PROCEDURE DATE: Apr 21 2014

INTERPRETATION: CT angiography of the circle of Willis and neck, brain CT

CLINICAL INDICATION: Subarachnoid hemorrhage
TECHNIQUE: Direct axial CT scanning of the circle of Willis and neck was obtained from the vertex to the level of the clavicular heads after the dynamic intravenous injection of 90 cc of contrast. Sagittal and coronal maximum intensity projection reformats were provided.
COMPARISON: Brain CT dated 04/21/2014
FINDINGS: There is extensive subarachnoid hemorrhage filling the basal cisterns and extending into the sylvian fissures bilaterally. There is mild hydrocephalus. Ventricular size has increased minimally compared with the prior study. No intraparenchymal hemorrhages identified. Interventricular hemorrhage is again noted within the third and lateral ventricles.

Evaluation of the circle of Willis demonstrates a basilar tip artery measuring approximately 1.7 mm at the base of the aneurysm. Height of an aneurysm is approximately 3 mm. No other areas suspicious for aneurysm are identified.

IMPRESSION: Basilar tip aneurysm measuring roughly 1.7 mm at base.

Extensive subarachnoid hemorrhage predominantly within the basilar cisterns and extending into the sylvian fissures bilaterally.

Mild hydrocephalus which is minimally increased compared with prior study dated 04/21/2014 at 6:50 a.m.

In the early afternoon, I asked one of Holly's friends, Christy, if she could solicit letters from Holly's friends and colleagues. I wanted to read these aloud at Holly's bedside once I was allowed to see her. I did not know if Holly would be conscious, but I hoped her brain could somehow process these notes of love and support on some level.

Christy's e-mail to friends and colleagues at Drew University, where Holly had earned her doctorate:

Date: Mon, Apr 21, 2014, 4:32 p.m.
Subject: Holly Hillgardner

To the friends and loved ones of Holly,

I am sorry to relay this news via e-mail. But I have just received a phone call from Greg Payan, who is Holly's boyfriend. Apparently, Holly had a brain aneurysm this morning and is in very critical condition. She is currently at Manhasset Hospital in Long Island and Greg is with her, as well as a number of family members. She is going to be in surgery tomorrow morning, and the surgery is very risky. Greg is asking for prayers for Holly and the surgery.

Additionally, if you would like, Greg has asked for letters from people who care about Holly to express your care for her. He plans to read these out loud to her before she goes into surgery. If you would like to send a letter for her, please e-mail it to Greg. Sometime tonight would be good, so that he can have them before surgery in the morning.

Greg specifically asked for prayers from the Drew community during this time.

Please feel free to call, text, or e-mail if you have any questions. I'll be in touch with Greg and can relay news as I hear anything.

Once Christy hit the send button, notes began to flood into my phone from Holly's Drew community. Soon after, I began to receive messages from my friends, her friends, and many of her former students from Texas as the word spread. Many of these notes are excerpted throughout the pages that follow.

Nancy e-mailed:
Greg,

I just got an e-mail from Dee Dee about Holly, and I'm just beside myself. Please know my thoughts are with you and Holly's sister. All my strength goes to Hol. Please tell her I love her and to hang in there. Her beauty and goodness and light are shining even while she's fighting. I'll be praying and sending all the positive vibes I can muster to all of you.

Neese e-mailed:
Holy Sweet Jesus, Greg,

I just got the news from Brian. I pray to God that Holly will be OK. You tell Holly this is bullshit and unfair. Tell her that she's a fabulous and strong woman. Tell her that her strength will make her pull through this with flying colors. Tell her there are too many people who love her, and this is the only option she has. Please tell her I am praying for her and for you.

I love you, honey. Be strong. Let me know if you need anything, anything at all.

Catherine e-mailed:
o god, greg.
  No words yet.
  Wish we could surround you both now with miraculous healing force.
  We will do our damnedest.
  And she is a miraculous being.
  Yes, praying.

Karen e-mailed:
Hi Greg,

I'm with Christy now. I'm so, so sorry this is happening and so grateful you were there. And so grateful I had the time to laugh and reflect with you both last night at dinner. I wrote something to Holly below. I want to say so much more but want to send my thoughts as soon as possible. I love Holly with all of my heart and am praying with all of my soul. I will always be here for you both.

Much love and in deep prayer.

<u>Please read this to her:</u>
Dearest Holly,

There are not enough words to express what you mean to me. As our friendship has deepened, my respect and love for you has grown exponentially. I love you so, so much. I look up to you and admire the compassion and care and confidence and support you bring to all you do. Your laughter and wit and smile and all that you are in a room makes every bit of the day one is with you better.

My work would not be the same without you, but more importantly, I would not be the same without you. Knowing you has made me a better woman, friend, colleague, partner, scholar, and teacher. You and your friendship have been a teacher to me and to so many. Your life has brought a level of mattering and meaning to so many, and I don't have enough words to show how grateful I am.

Whether it was me freaking out about comps, or us talking through your dissertation as we walked on the beach, or talking about family, or sexying up conference papers, or just laughing and eating and drinking together, I have cherished and learned from every moment with you. I don't think there is a colleague I admire more.

You are a brave, fierce friend and a light in my life. While you go through this, know that I am willing all of my soul and energy and prayers to you. I would walk through fire if it would help you right now. I will always be there for you and love you, you beautiful, strong woman.

I love you so much.

Sam e-mailed:
Hi Greg,

Though we never met, from the way Holly talks about you, I sure wish that our paths had crossed while I lived up that way. Thanks for receiving these e-mails and know that you, too, are in a lot of prayers tonight.

Please Stay

Dear Holly,

We just got word about what you're going through and are heartbroken. You're in an awful lot of prayers this night and are right at the front of ours. You were a partner in snark and in trying to see the big picture during our doctoral years, and I eagerly await the time when we can crack open a beer and talk about how insane it all was. Though I'm no good at correspondence, your friendship means a lot to me, and I always learn of your adventures with a twinge of envy and admiration. A whole lot of people love you, and they've all got it right. Hang in there. Peace.

Holly's friend John posted about her on Facebook:

John
April 21, 2014 · Edited

Please keep my friend Holly Hillgardner in your thoughts. She is one of the sweetest people I know- young, energetic, full of life, always smiling and best friends with a lot of my close friends, a good member of the community, a yoga instructor who really gets engaged with the students,, and a solid member of the community. She is only in her 30's and had an aneurysm today and will have emergency surgery tomorrow morning.

Happy thoughts, Holly. Pull fucking through and fight. God damnit. Fight.

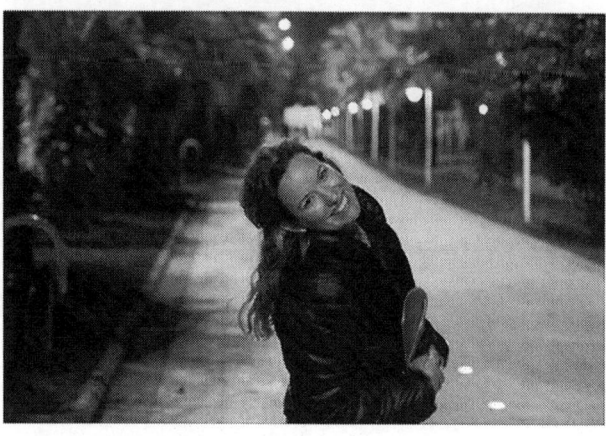

👍 Like   💬 Comment   ↗ Share

Michelle e-mailed:
Greg,

I am at a loss for words. I wish I were there to hug you and support you through this trying time. I am sending thoughts, prayers, and healing energies to Holly now.

Dee said that you would read a note to Holly. If you could, I would appreciate it. Please kiss her for me. Love to you.

Holly,

My dear friend, I hoped our next beach conversation would have included you next to me celebrating your love and happiness. There are so few people that we meet and have beautiful connections and friendships with. The times we spent together are precious. Even with me disappearing off the grid constantly, every time I hear your voice or see you, it is as if no time has passed at all. Thank you for being my constant and true friend. Now, while you rest, I hold you in my thoughts and prayers. Be strong and be brave. Know that you are surrounded by love and light.

Laurel e-mailed:
Holly,

I have always enjoyed your company as we navigated the Drew program together. The qualities that have struck me will help guide you in this very difficult time. You have always conveyed a sense of joy and calmness and a quality of centeredness that underlies both. As you go into this surgery, know that you are strong and have deep strengths within you to help you through this. Tap into that centeredness, that calm sense of self and confidence, and all the joy and warmth that you have given to others. Let your body be calm and send its energies toward your healing. I will be holding you in the light, as we Quakers say, sending my life energies and prayers in your direction, praying that the God that is all around us in this life surrounds you with light and life and a strength that you didn't realize was there.

My colleague Rachael e-mailed:
Dear Holly,

I have only met you twice, and this last Friday was the second time. Even though our meetings have been brief, I feel like I know you so well. Greg is fantastic with keeping us all updated with the great things in his life outside of the office. I know you to be such a smart, vibrant woman. You are always on an adventure around the world, exploring faraway lands as well as your own internal landscapes. I find that to be so admirable. You are such a warm and strong soul. I know you will get through this hiccup in life with a healthy recovery. Both you and Greg still have a lot of living to do together. There are many more mountains to climb, places to see, and memories to make. My love and thoughts are with you right now. Thank you for the opportunity to know you as the beautiful person that you are and to remind us all how to live better and fulfilling lives. We will all be so happy to see you soon. Lots of love to you, Holly.

P.S. Greg, I just want you to know that we all love you so very much! We are here for you and understand what a devastation this is. Be positive! These hard times are a testament to our ability to overcome struggle with love and grace. Holly will come out of this 100 percent! Please let us know how you are and if you need anything, day or night.

Wanda e-mailed:
My dearest Holly,

You are a dear soul sister to me…I love you and am praying for you to pull out of your coma…The world is a better place with you in it.

You and Greg have inspired me to hold on to the dream of true love.

I love you, my dear Holly…Can't wait to see you soon.

You have a beautiful, amazing spirit.

If you feel divinely inspired to transition on your journey, know you are loved by many…

As I look back on the e-mail above, it stands out from so many others I received, because it was the only one to broach the possibility of Holly's death. Holly's friend Wanda is spectacular. She's a free spirit and loyal and a healer. As I look back on this note, I see Wanda's faith. It was as if Wanda understood on a deeper level than many of us that if Holly's life were to end, it would end surrounded by the love of those who knew her from around the world and that it was OK.

Tanya e-mailed:
Dear Greg,

Thank you for offering us this gift, this chance to send our prayers and wishes for healing and hopefulness for Holly and for all of you who stand with her in this difficult moment.

Holly,

You are in a place where wise and wonderful people bring you their finely tuned practice of medicine, and better yet, you are surrounded by your loved ones, who stand in courage and love with you. In a season of miracles in our faith traditions, we know that goodness happens and with reliability and regularity. We believe in your strength, joined with the expertise of your physicians, and the love of your family, friends, loved ones, and this Drew community that is standing in solidarity with all of you now. All things are possible. Peace and blessings.

Christy e-mailed:
Holly,

The first interaction that I had with you was at one of my first academic conferences. We were introduced, and I liked you right away. I remember thinking of how confident and happy you were, especially in an academic setting, which often makes me feel out of place. But you made me feel comfortable, and we easily talked at that first meeting like we were old friends. I remember seeing you on the train on the way back to the city and us riding beside each other, talking the whole time. You were so easy to talk to that I found myself revealing stories and things about myself that I would not normally tell someone who I just met. But you have the ability to make everyone around you feel comfortable, and so I opened up to you so easily. Holly, I want you to know how much you mean to me and how important your friendship is to me. You are such an inspiration to me (have I told you that I use that mug you got me inscribed with "WRITE LIKE A MOTHERF*CKER" whenever I spend time writing my dissertation?), and your encouragement has been such an influence in my life. Just hearing this past week about your book and your plans for your research is so exciting—you have such a passion for knowledge and teaching!

I love you dearly, and I want you to know that I am thinking of you, praying for you, and supporting you right now. I am by your side, holding your hand, and sending thoughts your way. You are one of my closest friends, and I am so grateful that we met.

Thinking of you, praying for you, holding you in my thoughts and prayers, xoxoxox (as you always sign your texts and e-mails).

We were getting little information from the medical staff, aside from the news that they were still trying to stabilize Holly. During the interminable hours in the waiting room, doctors occasionally asked us questions, but we received few answers as to why this happened—mostly because there were no answers.

Holly was not "at risk" for an aneurysm based on her age or lifestyle; an aneurysm at her age was a cruel genetic curse. The fact that it had ruptured was just terrible luck. Holly's nurse promised to update us once Holly was stable and before he left for the day. He came back around 9:30 p.m., a few hours after his shift was scheduled to end. He informed us that, at one point, the doctors had considered operating to fix the aneurysm the following day, but now they thought the surgery would put her at even greater risk, because her heart and lungs had been damaged during the bleed. She would have surgery as soon as they felt her heart and lungs could handle the anesthesia and surgery.

We were able to go into her room before leaving the hospital that evening, but she was unconscious and had a breathing tube down her throat. After talking to her for a few moments, we were told to go home, rest, and return in the morning. I left my contact information with the ICU staff, should they need to reach me. Of course, I knew any call might be my worst nightmare.

Word had spread about the surgery that was supposed to happen the next day, and even though it had been postponed, more and more e-mails arrived for me to read to Holly.

Catherine e-mailed:
Greg,
 A note for Holly is attached. I am grateful for the opportunity.
 Love and courage to you.

Holly, Holly, Holly.
 This is Catherine speaking to you. Please stay with us. Holly, as your teacher and, if I may presume, your mentor, I am with you this morning and somehow always.
 You have realized so much already, brought so much to fruition in your life. You have given exorbitantly to so many students, high school and now college. You have been such a joy and support to your friends. And there are so many future students awaiting your inspiration and guidance.
 And Holly, you have written a work of great import, wisdom, and beauty. I am embarrassingly proud of your *Passionate Nonattachment*. It must be published; it will be. It has a brilliance, traveling across scholarly and student audiences with amazing clarity. It is a significant contribution to the field of comparative theology. But Holly, it wants your finishing touches. And it wants the follow-up of all your future writings.
 Please stay.
 And so for me, Holly, you just helped me last week fill in missing bits and fix problems in my book. You were your utterly gracious self, offering me meticulous scholarly aid.

It was about Hadewijch and this poem:

In the Infinite
I reach
for the Uncreated
I have touched it,
it undoes me
wider than wide
Everything else
is too narrow
You know this well,
you who are also there.

Holly, I love you very much always. CK

Cynthia e-mailed:
Hi Greg,

It's probably some eight hours after I spoke to you, and I'm still sitting here in shock. It doesn't even seem real. I know that after everything you have gone through today, it must seem all too horrifyingly real. I wish I had some piece of consolation or something to say to you—but I don't. The only thing I can say and that I hope you already know is that I love you and Holly both very much and will be praying for her. If positive mental energies count for something, and I think they do, believe me, I will be doing my part to get our Holly back whole again.

If you could read this to Holly tomorrow, I would really appreciate it. I love that you are doing this, by the way.

Holly,

This is not a request or a plea, but rather an order that you get through this and get well. You make me laugh, you make me cry, you make me ponder all things about life, and you do this even before we start pouring our first glass of red wine. I suppose there are a million reasons why I treasure my friendship with you, but maybe none so much as the fact that you, Holly Hillgardner, inspire me. You inspire me to be kind and to giggle more. You inspire me to dance, and you inspire me to do better in this world. You inspire me to have another glass of wine, and you inspire me to use my brain more. Through the way you gently move in this world, you inspire…and inch me just a little step closer to the person I strive to be. So you're not going anywhere on my watch, my friend, because I need you here. Greg needs you here. Your family needs you here. We all need you here. Ruben and I will be praying for you. Although my heart aches for you right now, I'm going to channel all of that ache into positive and beautiful energies and will send it tomorrow while you are in surgery. I love you, my dear, sweet friend—so very, very much.

Demy e-mailed:
Hi Greg,

This is my letter for Holly. I am thinking of Holly and of you. Please let me know if you or Holly's sis need anything at all! I am praying for her.

To my dear and wonderful friend Holly,

I am sitting here trying to formulate the words, trying to organize my thoughts as I write this letter to you. How do I capture and tell you what an incredible and wonderful friend you are to me and what you mean to me? This day has been beyond surreal, and I am in shock thinking that this is happening to you. When I think of you, I think of your bright smile, with your bouncy golden hair, trendy accessories and jewelry, fabulous shoes, and super fashionable bag busting at the seams, laughing that wonderful hearty laugh from the bottom of your stomach, and your zest for new experiences. I cannot imagine what you are thinking or feeling right now. And all I can hope for is that you are feeling all our love, thoughts, and prayers, and that we are all here with you.

Since we found each other and became *true* and real friends, you have never let me down. I know who you are, and I feel that you accept and know me for who I am. I love that you see me and laugh at me (and with me) and that I can laugh at you and with you. I love the Holly-isms and quirks—and I love that you are so smart and brilliant. I have never met anyone who can get so much information from the different blogs and discussion boards. I love that sometimes you are scattered and may forget to buy a return trip back to West Virginia (OK, it only happened once) after a New York City visit, but you figure it out. I adore that you are truly so free-spirited and full of life that you embrace everything in your life and seek out everything that is offered to you. You take it all in and live it all to the fullest. One of my most favorite Hollyisms is that your trips revolve around food. I love that when I asked about Paris, the first thing you told me was about the food! And who goes to Turkey in search of anchovies along the Black Sea? Holly, of course. That is really the essence of who you are—and that makes me feel so very special that someone who is so amazing and seeks out so many incredible and inspiring experiences in life would stop and pick *me* as her friend.

I think of you tonight. My friend, I am so honored and appreciative you are in my life. I love you and am thinking of you.

Inge e-mailed:
Dearest Greg,

Count on my thoughts and prayers from Paris. I'll light a candle for Holly today at the Basilica of Sacre Coeur.

Jake e-mailed:
Greg,

It's pretty late, but I'm writing for both me and my partner, William. I'm devastated by this, so it's taken me a while to think of anything to say. I can't imagine what it's like for you and know we're thinking of you, too. I'm praying fiercely now. I send you this letter for reading to her for encouragement, hope, and strength.

Holly,

I'm sending you my love and prayers from Minnesota and love from William in Kenya as well. I can't tell you what a privilege it is to be your friend—my gratitude for all of our laughter, conversations, our classes together, our collective joking around, our beautiful dance parties in New York City at the Pyramid Club, and all of our conversations when I get to see you at the American Academy of Religion conference. You are by far the person I look forward to seeing the most at these things, because I know that you take them with a grain of salt, your humor, your beautiful laugh, and your characteristic compassion and laid-back joy.

I was thinking back to when we were able to sit down at AAR last year and catch up and celebrate your new job and finishing the defense and just all of the joy and happiness you were feeling then—the thrill of being finished, of resting in the joy of the moment. You referred to yourself as a West Virginia "mountain mama" at some point. And I laughed so hard. And then you sent me a Facebook message in February to tell me you had gotten your diploma in the mail. "Egads!" was all it read. And I laughed and celebrated.

Holly, I'm keeping this short because I know others want to say just as much. But we love you. I love you. I can't imagine the last crazy five years of this damn PhD program without you and your joy, your compassion, your care. We love you. I love you. And we're with you every step of the way.

With every single, hopeful fiber of my being, my deepest love for you, my dear Holly.

Sara e-mailed:
Dearest Holly,

Before I heard that you were in the hospital, in surgery, I had been thinking of you all day. You would laugh if I told you how I started thinking of you. I was reading a book about a woman's pilgrimage to India. But you would smile at the end of my story of my thoughts about you. My thoughts wandered to when we were staying together in the dorm at Drew during a conference, remember? We were so tired—we had been up many nights with guests and at parties—but we stayed up even longer talking, pouring our hearts out across those twin beds in that tiny room. You told me things close to your heart, of your grief, of how finding yoga got you through and gave you life again. I had used yoga as a similar salvation vehicle, but you had received the gift so much more completely. You had given it your whole heart. Because that is how you are, who you are. I think that night of talking endeared us to each other, and today as I was thinking back on it, it made me long to fly across the country and spend another night talking. I thought about how you give your heart to so much—your work, and your students, and Greg, and your family, and your practice. You show me what true devotion looks like, while staying strong in yourself, in your smile, with your feet always on the ground.

Later in the day, inspired by India, maybe, and by my thoughts of you, I was listening to my favorite devotional musician, Snatam Kaur. Have you heard of her? She is a Sikh. One song was so beautiful; I had not heard it before. It is about giving your soul to one path. It is called "Kabir's Song." At the end, she sings to her soul. She says:

Oh my Soul…
Breathe my Love
Breathe my Love
Breathe in the quiet center.

Then I got news that you are in the hospital, and so I send this message to you, Holly, to your soul, to your heart.

You have touched me, Holly, and so many people. Let your soul now sing to itself and to your body. Breathe in the quiet center. You have devoted yourself to seeking that place, and you can be there now, in a place of healing.

My soul goes out to you, Holly, and to Greg especially, with you now. May you both feel the love of all those who surround you near and far.

My parents have a guest room with a nice bed in their house, but I chose to stay on their couch. I knew I would barely be able to sleep, so I thought it best to have a few glasses of wine and watch some TV to distract my mind until some restless sleep overtook me that night. I kept seeing Holly—eyes closed in a room of so many machines and with a breathing tube down her throat. Just twenty-four hours earlier, we'd been watching television. I'd rubbed her feet, which had been draped across my lap in our usual spots as we lay on our couch. It had been happy and beautiful and peaceful and mundane....and it seemed like an eternity ago.

I could take little comfort that she was alive at day's end, even though that small victory was amazing unto itself. I'd made a conscious decision from the moment I arrived in the Neuro ICU waiting room that I would not look up what she was going through online. I chose to inform myself as little as possible, trusting that the doctors would inform me of anything I needed to know in this process. I had worked myself up in the past over mild mystery ailments on the Internet, coming away thinking I was going to die. I felt the less I knew about her long odds, the better. I knew the situation was still dire and that death was still a very distinct possibility. I did not need the Internet to remind me of that.

In the summer of 2013, Holly had been finishing up her PhD and writing her dissertation. This endeavor requires an insane amount of work. Most "normal" people pursuing this academic route cut off friends and family on some level and work countless hours in their university library, constantly on the verge of a nervous breakdown until the work is complete. This was totally unacceptable to Holly, as it would mean she would not be able to travel that summer. As a result, we conceived the Lobster Tour. I planned a nine-day trip through New England, strategically timed for just when Holly was most insane with work and needing to get out of the city before she lost her mind. She would bring her books and computer. Holly would work while I drove, and she would work some more in our hotel room each morning, her books sprawled out over our bed as I brought her coffee and breakfast. She worked more still when we would stop for a midday coffee break en route to our next destination. The plan was to go to two restaurants in each town, consume a lobster or lobster roll at one of the two stops, and then drive to the next town the following day. Holly ate, drank, and worked her ass off, and the result was a great dissertation and defense, passed with distinction, that would soon after be published as a book.

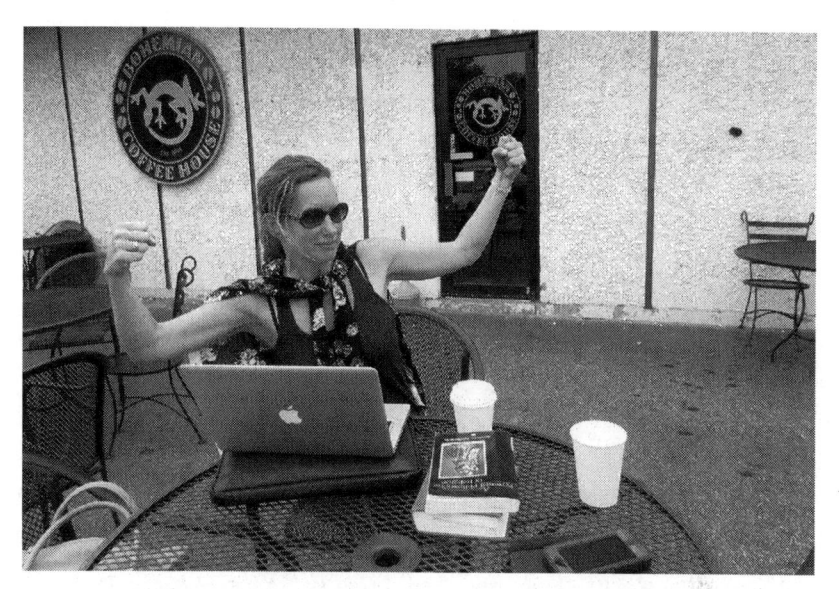

A dissertation/coffee break during the Lobster Tour.

This is how Holly lived her life. If her life was to end at thirty-nine, we had lived every bit of it. We had loved, laughed, eaten, drank, and given all we had to each day and to each other. She squeezed as much as she possibly could have from those thirty-nine years, and I considered myself incredibly blessed to have been with her for the last ten of them. It was some consolation, but it was not enough to find any sort of peace that night.

As time passed and the early morning hours of Tuesday arrived, I went to my phone to look at pictures of Holly and text messages I'd received over the last few days. It was a pale attempt to try and revisit the last few weeks, when things hadn't been as they were now. And knowing I'd left her unconscious with a breathing tube down her throat, I thought about hearing her voice. I looked through some old voice mails. I checked the dates and tried to think what we were doing each day the voice mails were archived to determine if each message would make me happy. I would scroll through, contemplate pressing the play icon, and then not do so. I did this for some time, trying to figure out if hitting 'play' would make me feel better or worse. In the end, I decided against it. If I wanted to hear her, she would need to be the one speaking to me. And if she did not make it through, I was sure I'd reconsider. But in that moment, my hope was that the next time I heard her, it would be her voice speaking to me—not a recorded message.

Dozens of random thoughts ran through my head when I turned off the lights, illuminated only by the dim glow of the TV. I thought about Holly and whether she would die. I ran through my head a list of "last times." The last time we'd gone out to dinner. The last time we'd kissed. The last time we'd checked in to a hotel in a foreign land. The last time we'd had sex. The last time we'd read the Sunday Times together. I tried to conceptualize my life without her, projecting out six months, projecting out twelve months, and I just could not do it.

I was consumed by thoughts of Holly dying. Could I potentially be planning her funeral shortly? I thought about the possibility of giving a eulogy for her in the next few days. I thought about scattering her ashes at sea, as she had requested in her will. And then I thought about a famous Johnny Cash quote. When interviewed some years ago, he'd been asked to define "paradise." Johnny had responded, "This morning, with her, having coffee."

His response had always moved me. It had only been a day, but I already missed my best friend. I would give anything in the world to wake up tomorrow and have a coffee with her and pretend this nightmare had never happened.

DAY 2—WAITING
April 22, 2014

I SLEPT FOR MAYBE AN hour or two overnight on my parents' couch, the phone next to my head. I was able to eat a bit, but I ate quickly, as I did through this whole ordeal. It was as if the only reason I was eating was to take in nutrients. Food had no flavor; it was just a means to an end—to give me energy and keep me going.

I arrived at the hospital early to find Holly with a breathing tube still down her throat, but now she was semiconscious and scared. She was heavily sedated, and when her eyes would open briefly, they would dart around the room, and she would move her lips and bite on the breathing tube as if trying to speak. Then she would nod off again. Holly's nurses' advice was to let Holly rest and try to prevent her from getting excited. The fact that she was having moments of consciousness and awareness of people in her room was a "great sign," according to the nurses.

7:33 a.m.
Shar texted me:
We are getting stuck at every train crossing.
We will be there soon.
Any news?

I replied:
With her. She's doing good.
Come in when u get here. Just you.
Still don't want her to have too much stimulation.

Shar texted:
OK, sounds good. Love you.

I replied:
I asked her to blink twice if she loved me, and she did.
Brain is working.

Shar texted:
WOW!

I replied:
Very sweet nurse today. Hunted me down.
Asked if I was fiancé and greeted me with smile.
Said she's doing great.

Kimberly e-mailed:
Holly,

I drove Route 2 this morning, a would-be shaman, searching the river for words to heal you. But the river did not speak. It just flowed on to the sea, and there you are in my mind's eye. You push out away from the breaking shoreline. You turn back, rise up on your board, and ride the wave back home to us. We love you, Holly! Get well. Come home.

Brooke e-mailed:
Good morning, Greg.

We are all feeling very hopeful this morning. I'll be sharing with you some of the messages from faculty and students throughout the day. One of Holly's students is organizing a card signing for her on campus today, and I'll be working with our club members to plan a prayer and poetry service for Holly. We'll have selections from all the major world traditions, including Mirabai. If you can, please let me know what room they'll be moving her to.

So many folks wanting to know what they can send, but I assume we'll need to wait until after the surgery.

Kap e-mailed:
Greg,

You don't know me—we may have met once—but I am a colleague of Holly's here at Bethany. I was deeply shocked to hear of what happened, and I just wanted you to know that my wife, Stephanie, and I are keeping her and you in our thoughts. Harald and Brooke are keeping us updated, but if there is anything I can do to help, please don't hesitate to ask. Working with Holly over the past few years has been sheer delight, and I have often said to my colleagues that she is exactly the kind of dedicated, sensitive, accomplished faculty member we need at this place—now more than ever. Again, know that our thoughts are with you as you await the outcome of the surgery and beyond.

HH e-mailed:
Hi Greg and Holly.

Sending y'all all kinds of love and hugs and prayers. I drove down Tulip Drive this morning and thought about how crazy it is that I live in the neighborhood where you grew up, Holly. It makes me think that if my boys grow up in the same neighborhood, they might turn out to be as amazing as you are. I am not sure how attending a workshop with you all those years ago landed me the most loyal of friends, but I am so grateful. Two girls named Holly, professors with PhDs. How funny life can be. You have been on my mind this last month, and I keep thinking about standing in your kitchen when you told me about first meeting Greg…I thought how much you deserved to be that excited about someone. I keep thinking about you surprising me for a wedding shower. I keep thinking about our last "holly-day" in Austin, where you finally decided that you "might have romanticized the Texas summer a bit." I have been madly in love with you since the moment we met and had lunch together at that workshop. It is a fierce sister love, and I am sending it across the country full blast today.

Greg,

I love you for being there for my girl when I can't. Not just today but always. I will jump on a plane in a New York minute. No matter what you both need. Just say the word. Holly, I love you. I am anxious to talk once your body heals. Love, prayers, happy thoughts…all on their way. I love you.

10:55 a.m.
Shar texted:
I don't want her to be alone.
Could you come back in once you eat,
if you can, so I can take a short break?

That morning, I sent my first e-mail update on Holly's condition to about twenty people. The list quickly grew to more than one hundred.

From:	**Payan, Gregory**
Sent:	**Tuesday, April 22, 2014, 11:03 a.m.**
Subject:	**Holly Update**

Mostly good news so far today. She recognizes me. She's sedated but opened her eyes when she heard my voice. Told her it will all be OK and to relax and stroked her cheek. Asked her to blink twice if she loved me and got two blinks. Awesome, awesome. She cannot talk, as she has a breathing tube. The not so good: her lungs and heart function were compromised by the bleed, and doctors don't want to do the procedure to fix the aneurysm until

they improve. The procedure is dangerous and has potential serious complications. Neurological signs are great now, but doctors have yet to go in to fix the aneurysm that is in such a bad spot. She is in good hands, and the head MD says the neurological-function news is great. That alone makes the heart and lung issues, which they think are temporary, worth it. While there is a chance it could bleed again, they feel that risk (based on other stable vitals and her resting) is minimal but still possible. A second bleed would be a disaster. Today is likely just a maintenance day, keeping her calm and quiet. Hoping lungs and heart improve so they can do procedure soon—tomorrow or Thursday. Thanks, all, for the thoughts and prayers and notes. They mean a lot. Forward to anyone I left out.

Elisabeth e-mailed:
I'm telling you she's going to be OK. Great news.

Later in the morning, I was out of the room, but Sharley was with Holly when she signaled for a pen and paper.

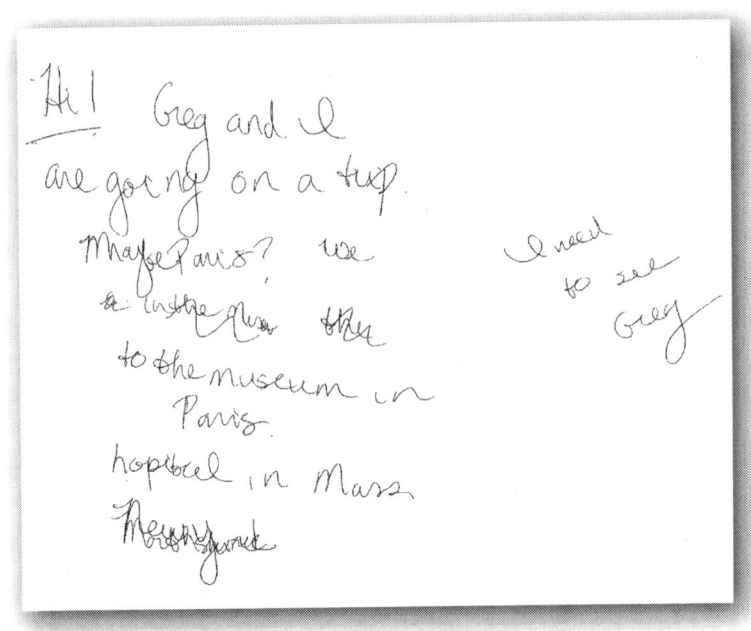

Holly tried to orient herself in her first note after regaining consciousness and asked to see me.

Holly could not talk due to her breathing tube and was obviously confused but trying to figure things out. She must have thought she was in Massachusetts, where her sister lives, as she woke up in unfamiliar surroundings and saw Sharley. It was her handwriting, in spite of the many drugs she was being given and just twenty-four hours after a severe brain hemorrhage. It was my first glimmer of hope that Holly was still in there.

When I returned to her room, I gave her a kiss and did my best to calm her down. She must have been terrified and confused to wake up in a hospital room with a tube down her throat, hooked up to machines, and with her hands tied down. (The staff feared Holly may try to pull out any lines attached to her.)

The hospital staff encouraged us to tell her what had happened and where she was, while trying not to scare her. Holly initially thought she was dying. Then, after learning she'd had a brain bleed, she began teasing me about not remembering my name. Her sense of humor was still there too! Once she understood that she had a brain hemorrhage that needed to be fixed, she immediately wanted the

Please Stay

doctors to know that she has a doctorate, which I could only assume meant that she wanted them to be very careful with her brain, whatever they chose to do regarding treatment.

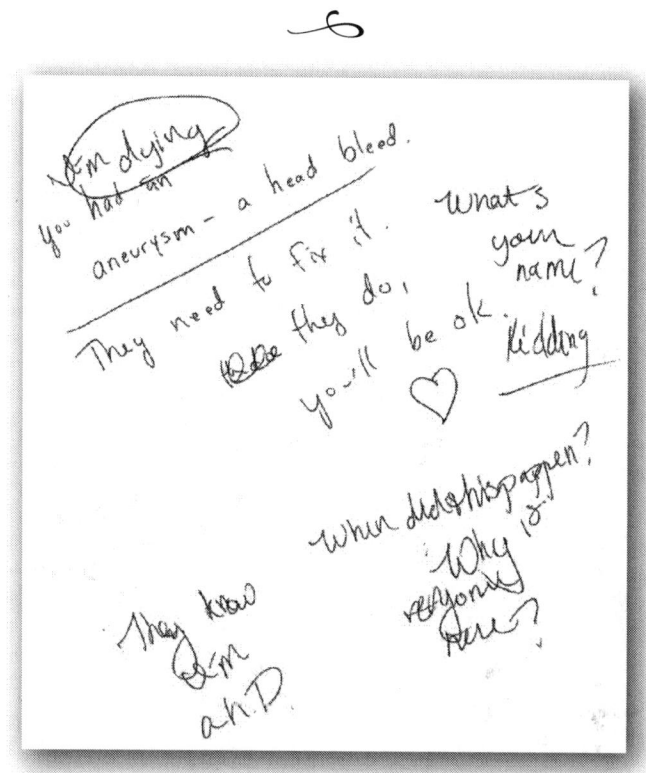

***

> I'm dying
> You had an aneurysm — a head bleed.
> They need to fix it.
> What will they do?
> What's your name?
> you'll be ok
> ♡
> kidding
> When did this happen?
> Why is everyone here?
> They know I'm a h.D.

This note shows her confusion and our back-and-forth communication. Holly wrote in script, while missing a few letters in her words understandably. I printed my replies.

***

Leila e-mailed:

Hi Greg,

First, I want to tell you that I just prayed to God to ask Him to help Holly fight for her life. She is such a strong woman—emotionally, mentally, physically, and spiritually. I asked Him to help her recover so that she

39

could continue to shine her light on others. I also asked Him to give you and all of her loved ones strength as you support her throughout her illness. It is so hard to watch someone you love suffer, and I know y'all need prayers as well.

Holly was my English II teacher at Arlington High School in 1998. She was the first teacher I remember who approached her job with energy, ambition, and a sincere passion for literature. On the first day of class, I knew things would be different because she wore a fitted gray suit, and she had springy honey-brown curls. "Who is this woman, and what is she thinking, looking so professional and cute in a public school?" I thought. She read aloud in a tone that showed she revered the text in her hands. She challenged us to dig deeper into an author's mind in a way that we had never been asked to before. She asked us what we thought about a piece of literature, and it was OK if we said that we didn't like it—we just needed to justify why. ;) She inspired me to come back to Arlington High School to teach English II. I'm wrapping up my ninth year, teaching a similar curriculum that she shared with me years ago. "Sharing" is the best way to describe her teaching philosophy—it was an exchange of ideas in a welcoming, respectful, challenging way, and I really appreciate that. Please tell Holly how much she has inspired me.

Becca e-mailed:
Hi Greg,

It's Becca. I don't even know how to start this e-mail…I'm so sad but hopeful. I wish I was there, and I'm so glad you are in her life and with her during this…all of the above…However, I do know that I want to say I am praying for you and Holly. Please let me know what I can do.

Below are the stories I would love you to read to her.

I loved driving down to Galveston to stay in her friend's house for the long weekend. We fell asleep on the beach one day and *fried* our skin! Mine was right on my bikini line, and I wanted to cry the whole way home it hurt so much! This trip was one of my favorites because we discussed Flannery O'Connor's short story. We talked about the characters, God, and the plot for about an hour. What I loved was that we were both so engaged in the conversation and discussing God, we didn't realize an hour had passed. Conversation is always so easy with us!

Toni Morrison's book *Paradise* is another one I love. We bought the book together and would exchange the book daily, reading only one chapter a night and discussing it the next day. Of course, Holly couldn't contain herself and would always read more than she should have. I love this about her though. I will read *Flight Behavior*, and we will have our book club in person soon!

I love that she gave pedicures to moms-to-be for their baby shower gifts. She loved to pamper them! Of course, the funniest story was when she was giving a woman the book *What to Expect When You're Expecting*. When we were walking to the baby shower, she realized she hadn't "un" dog-eared a part. I said, "Oh, did you find that at Half Price?" She said, "No, it is brand-new, but I read it first." I laughed soooo hard. Reading a pregnancy book? It was hilarious!

I love dancing in Dallas until the club closed! We looked forward to our holiday weekends so we could go and unwind on a Sunday night. We were always so tired and sweaty when we were on our way home at 2:30 a.m.

Mama's Pizza will never be the same for me. We had fourth-period conference and would go to lunch at 12:30 p.m. and eat the buffet. Yes, leave school early and not go back that day. :) The buffet ended at 2:30, so we would eat at 12:45 and then sit and talk until 2:15 and then eat again before we left. This is the place she told me she was going to Mexico to spend the summer that she met you, and this is the place she told me she was going to move to New York to be closer to you! I think of her every time I go in this place and wish she were with me to eat a double buffet again.

Even though she knows, please let her know I love her and that I am praying for all of you. Also, I would still love to come see her this summer!

Jenny e-mailed:
Ms. Hillgardner,

I remember you as a teacher, a mentor, and a friend. As a teenager, I always thought you were so beautiful, inside and out, and I hoped that one day

I could be as cool as I thought you were. When I was in high school, so much of my world was dark. I hadn't found my place yet. I had a few close friends, but I felt so different and alone in that school. Yet for some reason, being in your yoga class changed that for me in some small way. You introduced us to a whole new way of exercising and thinking. I shared mat space with the "preps" and "jocks" I once viewed as belonging to a different species. I started to realize that we are all the same at our core.

Probably the best memory I have, other than your friendly smiles and wise words, which were just what a black-clad teenage misfit needed, was of the time we went to a yoga studio in Fort Worth.

I had managed to complete a full yoga session (without skipping anything and retreating to child's pose) several times at school before we went. I remember you invited the whole class, and only several of us could go. I still remember how strong and happy I felt, practicing with you, my classmates, and other yogis I didn't know. At the end of the class, when it came time for reflection and closing, the instructor led us in an "ohm" that I felt in my very soul. I mean it. I could hear everyone's voice join together, and then I could feel the sound vibrating in my bones and blood, and it seemed like the sound came from everywhere at once and was much deeper and louder than a dozen human voices could accomplish.

Seriously, as cheesy as that sounds, that really happened. That's how I felt on our yoga field trip, that our ohm truly had the whole universe singing along. It may have just been physical exhaustion and excitement, or perhaps it was some sort of spiritual moment. Whatever the case, you were part of that memory, Ms. Hillgardner. I hate to think about you in a hospital bed, waiting to wake up, and I wonder what you're thinking or dreaming right now. I just know how strong and beautiful you are, and the world is a much better place with you in it. I know you can beat this. You're in my thoughts.

Michelle e-mailed:
Hey Greg,
Sending you love and hugs. I cannot imagine how you are doing right now. If you don't mind, I'd love to have you read her another note for me? I

feel her floating around. I keep on sending her healing love and prayers, but if I were there, I would babble these words to her and maybe play some quiet healing music. Please make sure someone is looking after you! If there is *anything* I can do, let me know.

And now, for Holly...

Hey, baby love! Sorry you have to hear my words in the lovely voice of Greg, but I have to work with the tool available to me. So I've been meditating and chanting and sending you all sorts of healing energies. I can feel you floating in the darkness...keep remembering the love all around you. Thinking of you while you are in this space of limbo. Thinking that you, my dear spiritual friend, seem to be in the perfect space to have an experiential understanding of all that you have been studying and practicing over these past years. So, my love, listen...I think we should have a good long talk about this when you are ready! I even had an image of you writing a book like Jill Bolte Taylor or that doctor who wrote *Proof of Heaven*. No pressure, but it seems like you are finally in a unique position to understand *it* all from a different perspective.

Now, in this state of rest, get strong; be still. Know that you are surrounded by so much love, light, and support. Love you!

Kandrea e-mailed:
Holly,

I know that you guys are receiving a lot of love from all over the nation right now, so I'll keep it short and sweet. I know that right now is a very hard time for you and your loved ones, but please stay positive and keep hope alive, because that's what you taught me and many others to do. From English projects to yoga classes, I still tell everyone about how much you mean to me and how you changed my life. While in high school, I gained a different perspective on the world and how to handle life, all through you. I don't think I have ever met another person with such a radiant and glowing spirit and the strong desire to help others. I live my life striving for the peace and grace that you possess. So please know that I and the rest of the world are standing behind you right now. We are all here to give back the many years of love that you gave us all so graciously.

So please don't fret. We are all by your side. A woman like you deserves to have the world stand around her, and we are all here, praying for a fast and complete recovery. Even if you don't remember me, I still love you with all of my heart. It was an honor to be in your presence, and I hope to be in it once again.

You are admired!
With *all* of the *love* I have, Kandrea
Devoted yoga and English student 2003–2005

From: Payan, Gregory
Sent: Tuesday, April 22, 2014, 8:31 p.m.
Subject: Holly Update

First off, there are a lot of people on this list. Be sure to reply just to me and not all. Thanks.

Thank you for all the e-mails I have received over the last two days. Holly is to all of us different things—a friend, a colleague, a professor, a sibling, a muse, a fiancée, or a soul mate—but to all of us she is the same: one of the most special people we have ever known or had the privilege to call friend.

It is Tuesday eve as I write this, and she is resting comfortably right now. She has a ruptured aneurysm yet to be repaired. That said, she is in no pain and is sleeping a lot. Please know that there may be someone I have left off this list. If that is the case, please forward this note. I can only apologize—trying to balance taking care of her, keeping people updated, and trying to fight through tears may result in some e-mail addresses that have not been cut and pasted. Please know that every last note is cherished. I have not yet read your beautiful notes to her. The doctor does not want her agitated, and she is resting. We just go in to hold her hand or scratch her head and tell her things will be OK. Conversations have been short, per the doctor's request. When we speak to her, she opens her eyes and tries to remove her tubes to talk. We just hold her whenever possible.

I will try to recap the whole set of incidents for those of you who have not heard. Some of this story is not happy, so feel free to jump to the next paragraph if this is hard for you to read. Holly woke up crying on Monday morning with the worst headache of her life. Within a few minutes, she began to convulse and gag, and I called 911. I held her until the EMTs arrived. She was taken to the closest hospital, where a scan showed an arterial bleed on her brain, and she was put in an ambulance to be transferred to where they specialize in treatment of such. She is currently at Long Island Jewish hospital in Manhasset, receiving excellent care. On the way to Manhasset, she stopped breathing in the ambulance and had to be intubated. When she arrived at the hospital, it was a dire situation. She was fifty-fifty to live, not responsive to stimuli, and unable to breathe on her own. I was seated with a social worker upon my arrival and asked if I needed a priest, once they informed me she may not make it. Brain hemorrhages are graded on a one-to-five scale, I to V, with V being as close to death as you can be on arrival. Holly was a IV. She had a drain inserted in her skull to relieve pressure on her brain and was stabilized over the next twelve hours.

Once diagnosed, it was determined she has a small aneurysm in a bad spot, and it bled throughout her skull. "Valuable real estate," as her doctor said when describing the area. There are two ways to treat it, and the doctors told us what they felt was best. Her sister and I were in agreement. She will undergo a "coil" procedure, as opposed to going in and putting a clip on it. In the "coil" procedure, thin platinum coils are packed into the aneurysm to prevent blood from flowing in. A "clipping" would involve opening Holly's skull to place a clip over the aneurysm to prevent blood from flowing in. It is extremely dangerous and much more invasive than the "coiling."

Most of yesterday was spent stabilizing Holly. Surprisingly, when we left last night, she was already showing small signs of improvement neurologically and was raising her arms and legs on command. We left last night hopeful, trying to get some rest, as today there was going to be a dangerous surgery to fix the aneurysm. They did not want to do it yesterday, as there had already been too much trauma to the area.

Holly's sister and I arrived this morning to mostly good news. Her functioning was continuing to improve, but her heart and lungs were temporarily damaged due to the bleed. Surgery was put off until tomorrow, maybe Thursday. Today saw continued neurological improvement and improvement to her lungs. Holly currently sleeps fifty-nine minutes of every hour. She wakes up a bit startled but calms down quickly. She recognizes me and others, but she has a tube down her throat and cannot yet speak. I talked to her first thing this morning, and she nodded when I asked if she knew I loved her. She nodded when I asked her if she knew she'd be all right. I asked her to blink twice if she loved me, and she blinked twice. (Remember, she's still intubated, so blinking is how we know she understands, as she cannot speak.) These are amazing signs after what she went through twenty-four hours ago. She then fell back asleep. If you know and love Holly, this, too, is a good sign. Holly never passes up an opportunity to sleep, unless there's an early flight to catch to an exotic land.

Later in the morning, her sister was with her, and Holly motioned as if she wanted to write. She was given a pad and paper. She wrote "Hi!" to her sister…yes, with an exclamation point. She then was asked how she was, and she wrote, "Greg and I are planning a trip." (We had hoped to go to Italy). She then thought and got it wrong. "Paris, maybe? A museum in Paris?" We have been to Paris a few times, but not this trip plan. But again, great signs. She nodded when we asked if she knew she was in a hospital, and when she was asked where, she wrote "Massachusetts."

Again, not right, but a great guess, as her sister was beside the bed and she knew her sister lives in Massachusetts. When told New York, North Shore hospital, she wrote "North Shore." This is truly remarkable, and her handwriting...unmistakably Holly's—no difference at all. The rest of today, she has been resting peacefully, although she got pretty agitated when I said good night. Good agitated, if it matters, as she wanted to write some more and listen to me talk.

She remains sedated, and tomorrow will be a tough day. If the doctors feel she's OK, they will try to fix the aneurysm. It is a dangerous surgery. If all goes well tomorrow, she will remain in the hospital for a minimum of three more weeks while they monitor the area where the bleed was. She will be at an increased risk for a stroke in the area for some time and under constant supervision.

Today was a great day for hope and the power of collective prayer and good thoughts. I am grateful to all of you. I cannot wait to share the beautiful notes you all have sent when the doctors say I can read them to her. Our Holly is beautiful and smart and a fighter—and she has a fighting chance. She is under the best of care by a small army of doctors and nurses. She is fierce and in restraints, only because she is trying to remove her tubes when she wakes, stubborn as she is. As I told the nurse, this is a good sign, as she probably heard there were good waves in Montauk, and she wanted to catch a ride on her surfboard.

Tomorrow and the coming weeks will be hard. While today was great, there are many battles left to fight. I remain hopeful but scared. I am known in these parts for my red eyes and cry towel, which is used often and will remain draped over my shoulder until she is well. The thought of a world without her is something I, and all of you, just cannot bear. For all of you who know and love her, I promise to remain strong around her and share all the love and thoughts and prayers you have sent over the next few weeks, whenever I am by her side.

Many have asked about visiting or flowers. Flowers are not allowed in her room ever. Cards and photos will eventually be welcome, along with visitors. That time is not yet, but I will tell you when it is.

All of you, thank you for your collective love. It means the world to me, my family, Holly's family, and most of all, to her. She can feel it, and I look forward to the day when she can tell each one of you how wonderful you all were to her when she needed it most and got all the collective love that this group (and anyone mistakenly left off) could muster.

As the person who has been blessed to have this wonderful person as my life partner, I cannot express how much you all mean to me and to her. Holly's sister, who has been with me through the last few days, expresses her deepest appreciation as well. She has Holly's toughness and takes good care of me, too, when I falter.

Keep the thoughts coming and the prayers. Tomorrow (or Thursday) is a really critical day when she undergoes the procedure. I know I can count on you all for continued well wishes and thoughts across the miles.

Much love to all of you.

Karen e-mailed:

Greg,

Thank you for all you are doing. You too are fierce and wonderful, and our Holly is so lucky to have you. I can't even imagine all you are going through and juggling. Know that I am here for anything not only Holly needs, but that you need as well. Thank you for keeping me, through Christy and now this note, so informed. We are sharing the vital information with the Drew people who need it. Mainly, though, thank you. Truly, I will always be there for both you and Holly in any capacity and in particular over the next weeks and months. Please know you have me and Christy as additional family in New York City.

Lydia e-mailed:
Thank you, thank you, Greg. Just remember to change that cry towel every now and again.

Carol e-mailed:
Greg,
 I wish I could do more, but this is all I have…

A gift is pure when it is given from the heart,
to the right person at the right time
and at the right place,
and nothing is expected in return.
 —Bhagavad Gita

10:22 p.m.
I texted Shar:
Just called the ICU. She's doing good.
Her numbers are above the threshold
they were looking for on the cardiac test,
and as of now, she looks good for tomorrow a.m. surgery.
Things could change, but that's the current plan.
Nurse says she's doing great,
and I told him to tell her Greg and Shar love her.
Love you and see you tomorrow.

                                          Shar replied:
                        Wow, great! See you in the morning.
                            We are coming for 7:30 a.m.

Erin e-mailed:
Hi Greg,
 I don't expect you to remember me, because it's been quite a few years since we met, but I'm a good friend of Holly's from Arlington. Holly and I first met in 1998 in a book club that was started by Nancy, one of our college

professors. Then we taught at Arlington High School together for six years. In fact, Holly also officiated at my wedding in June of 2004, right before she flew to Mexico and met you.

Please know that Holly, you, and your families are in my thoughts and prayers constantly. I believe that Holly's beautiful stubbornness, her unfailing perseverance, and her incredible strength are going to see her through this. Please give her love and hugs from me, and keep the updates coming.

Marjorie e-mailed:
Hi Greg.

Demy sent me your e-mail update about Holly—I had seen thoughts and prayers on Facebook.

What shocking news—I can only imagine how difficult it must be for you and your families. I'm in Montauk right now and coincidentally was just thinking of you guys, wondering if you were planning to be out here.

You are such a warm, loving pair who truly "get" each other—I can't think of anyone who exudes more light than Holly! Please squeeze her hand from me.

Tomorrow I will be at the water, sending her warm wishes and lots of prayers. I can just see her smiling right now, surfing and smiling!

Amy e-mailed:
Hi Greg,

It's Amy, one of Holly's friends from high school. We've met a few times long ago (before I had kids). I live in New York.

This is just so unspeakably horrible. Keely and I were texting for an hour last night in an attempt not to panic. I wish we were there to hug you and keep you in fresh cry towels.

I'm sending as much positive energy her way as possible. If there's anyone who can recover from a brain aneurysm, it's Holly. She is so, so strong and such a ray of beautiful energy and light. No wonder she has a huge tribe of people who love her.

Did you ever hear how we met? We kinda met twice. When we were sophomores in high school, we heard about each other for months because people thought we were twins. And of course, I often heard about Holly, the poor girl whose mom just died of leukemia. We didn't officially meet until February at a mutual friend's birthday party. We got on like a house on fire. Soon we were having sleepovers and dancing to "Groove Is in the Heart."

It wasn't until a year later that we realized we had met years before, in sixth grade. Holly went to church camp with a friend, and I was at the same church camp. Toward the end of the week, we both had a falling out with our friends. So we sat next to each other on the bus ride home. We sang and laughed for the entire drive back to Arlington. Nowadays we would have exchanged cell numbers and e-mails, easily keeping up the friendship with the Internet. But it was 1986, and although we lived very close to each other, we didn't meet again until 1990.

I love her so much. She has been through two lifetimes of bad luck. She deserves to live past one hundred.

If you or Shar need anything, I am just across the sound in Larchmont, New York.

When Holly's friend recalls her bad luck in the above e-mail, she references a life Holly lived that was far from easy. Holly grew up in Arlington, Texas, and had a typical suburban upbringing with her parents and younger sister, but early in Holly's teenage years, her mother was diagnosed with leukemia. After battling the cancer for a few years, her mother succumbed. A single father coming to grips with his wife's death, running a business, and trying to parent two strong girls by himself raised Holly and Sharley the rest of their teenage years.

At twenty, Holly married her high school sweetheart, only to see him diagnosed with liver cancer just a few years later. Her husband, B. G., would die two years after his diagnosis. By her midtwenties, she had lost two of the most important people in her life.

In spite of the losses, Holly moved forward, determined to live every day to the fullest and never let herself be defined by such losses. Almost two decades after her late husband's death, she lamented the fact that when you Googled her, the first few results returned were about her being a widow. Holly adored her husband and will always love him, but she hated the fact that something like that would be one of the first things seen.

Most recently, her father, a good, kind man who did his absolute best raising two daughters as a single father after their mom's death, had developed a gambling problem exacerbated by dementia. He'd lost his home, his business, his savings, and his second wife. Holly and her sister had been trying to arrange his care on a daily basis for the past few years. He was not physically or emotionally capable of visiting Holly, or even talking to her as Holly remained in the ICU.

This was not a charmed life. It was a hard one. But one that was also filled with as much joy as she could squeeze out of it every day she walked the earth.

Megan e-mailed:
Hi Greg,

I got the update through Keely. Thanks for writing that; it must have been hard. I am so, *so* glad she was there with you. It kills me to think how terrified she must have been, and she is not easily scared. Please let her know I'm thinking of her (and not much else) and to please cut it out. Her Facebook page of travels used to make me so jealous; now it is depressing and occasionally infuriating.

Lloyd e-mailed:
Greg,

I only recently had the pleasure of meeting Holly last week when you brought her to the office. I came away from our brief conversation thinking that she had an amazing life force and just radiated positive energy. I even mentioned meeting her to my wife because she was so impressive.

Having just lost my father, I know the fear and concern that you must be feeling. Your e-mails have been an inspiration, and your strength and love can be such a powerful force for Holly's recovery.

In the late hours, as I tossed and turned on my parents' couch, I began to try to process what had happened. The first day, I had just been in shock about the suddenness and potentially life-ending consequences that I felt minute by minute. The second day, and for weeks after, it all seemed like a dream. Every day, usually en route to the hospital or returning home at day's end, at some point at a red light, I would clutch the steering wheel and, in utter frustration, think, "This cannot be happening. This fucking cannot be happening."

Now that it was clear this was going to be a reality for the upcoming weeks and months, I had to sort out my new life. Taking care of Holly was first and foremost in importance. Sharley and I would text daily and make sure someone was with Holly at the hospital from 8:00 a.m. to 10:00 p.m. Early on, there was a lot of overlap, but eventually we broke the days into shifts.

Shar also had to sort out her life. While her husband and small child had come down from Massachusetts with her on the day of the rupture, they returned home shortly thereafter. Shar stayed a few miles from the hospital with Holly's and her cousin, but soon, she would have to go home to her job, husband, and young son.

I would stay on my parents' couch for the foreseeable future. Work, for me, would not be an issue. I worked for a good company and had a great boss, who offered as much time as I needed. I would spend as much time at the hospital as I could, while still responding to work e-mails. If nothing else, that was a break from the daily hospital anxiety. I don't remember for sure, but I don't even think I put an "out of office" message on my e-mails. If I got an e-mail while Holly was in the ICU, I likely replied to it soon after. This kept me in the world and likely a bit saner than if the entirety of my world had revolved around the hospital walls for twelve to sixteen hours a day.

DAY 3 — THE COILING
April 23, 2014

<u>7:33 a.m.</u>
Shar texted me:
Morning. How is she?

I replied:
Give me five minutes.
They are giving Holly a quick exam.

Shar texted:
Take your time.

Shar arrived at the hospital shortly after our exchange, and Holly was prepped for surgery. Her heart and lung function were still not great, but the staff felt it was worth the risk to have the surgery. They felt they had to get rid of the aneurysm as soon as possible before it potentially ruptured again.

Emily e-mailed:
Greg,

I wrote Holly an e-mail last night but didn't send it to you, b/c I just can't fathom the idea of you reading it to her in a hospital bed. I've passed your update on to my friends who all know and love Holly, and every single one is holding her in the light at this moment.

Greg, please stay positive and know you are being held up by hundreds of people who love Holly and want to help you be strong for her.

I'll be waiting to hear as soon as she's out of surgery. Thinking of you both every minute and pulling for her with all my heart.

Catherine e-mailed:
Greg,

I am grateful we met at Holly's dissertation defense, so that I can visualize the scene and hear your voice.

Got today's message. I keep thinking of the fingers of brilliant surgeons. I keep trusting the miraculousness of our Holly.

Holly went into surgery midmorning. The coil procedure was supposed to take a few hours. I sat with my parents, watched TV, and e-mailed a few people. I had a sense of peace about the situation and was very hopeful. Unfortunately, my peace belied what was actually happening during surgery. Things were not going according to plan.

Brooke e-mailed:
Hi Greg,

I know you've gotten a ton of messages, but whenever she is awake and able to relax a bit after the surgery, I want you to read this to her.

Holly,

We have begun and ended this school year with some neurological nightmares, but we are survivors. You have scared the ever-loving shit out of me, but you are going to be fine—even better than before. I have already endured too many nights of bad TV without you now and am catching up on *Mad Men* for you. I am always picking my phone up to text you whatever annoying or funny thing I'm experiencing, but most of all I want to say, "Where the hell are you? I *need you*!" We are a dynamic duo here (and everywhere). People see us as family because we are. Everyone has been amazing, wanting to know how they can help, offering so many encouraging words, and most of all expressing their unending love and admiration for you. You've been here two years and are beyond ensconced, ingrained, and adored.

Your students have been gracious, patient, and concerned. You are beloved. They have been hugging me like they are hugging you vicariously, like you'll "get it" if they hug me, because they know how close we are. People have actually been asking me how I'm doing, as if that's a thing. I'll be fine if you're fine, and I'll be scared if you're scared, and I'll be in pain if you're in pain. I'll be there as soon as I can to hug you and bring you notes from students and friends. I'll bring a "get well" cake and sing the "get well" song from *Seinfeld*. Then we'll sneak some Petite Syrah and laugh about stupid lines from our site visit papers.

We are a department and a family with a whole bunch of unruly children to educate. *Refuah shleimah*, and I love you.

Summer e-mailed:
Hi Greg,

I got the news just now. Holly was my teacher at Arlington High School, and I wanted to share a few stories you could read to her.

Holly was my AP English teacher sophomore year of high school. I remember how she would walk into the classroom in the morning with a bounce in her step, just enough for her hair to bounce a little. Twice a week for a while, Holly would bring herself a treat from Starbucks—it appeared to be some sort of iced latte. After Holly settled in, she always smiled and brought such positive energy to the class.

Holly,

Your smile was contagious, and I am grateful for that. Not everyone was as excited for English class, but I was, because I had you as a teacher! I remember our final project that year—I can't remember what you called it, but it was a test of our knowledge of different rhetorical devices, where we read a novel and then proceeded to pick a theme and make our own storybook of poems, drawings, stories, and so on! It was probably one of the most challenging but fun projects I did that year!

Please Stay

I remember one day you came into class and told us a story about a woman who gave you some advice on a particularly frustrating day. The woman, I think, found you weeping in the bathroom, and she told you, "Honey, when life brings you lemons, add some water and sugar and make some lemonade!" I ad-libbed there, but you get the point! Your reaction to her response was so real and raw, and as an adult, I can relate now. You told us that you just didn't want to hear that, and why wasn't it OK in the moment just to be upset? We are all human! I will remember that forever.

Holly, you are such an inspiration to your students/yogis! I am sending you positive thoughts and love through these memories.

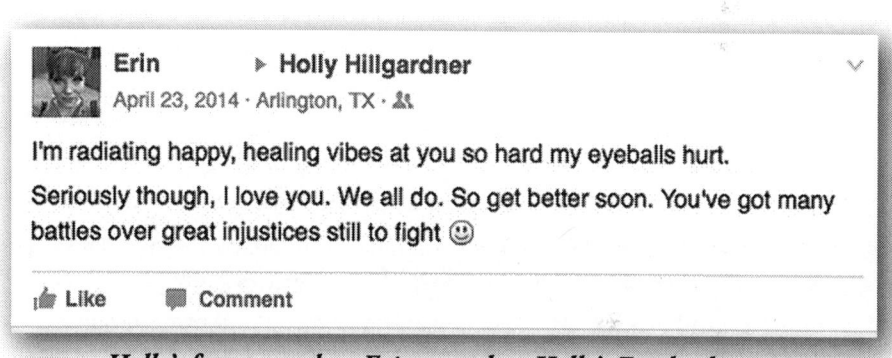

> **Erin** ▸ Holly Hillgardner
> April 23, 2014 · Arlington, TX
>
> I'm radiating happy, healing vibes at you so hard my eyeballs hurt.
> Seriously though, I love you. We all do. So get better soon. You've got many battles over great injustices still to fight 😊
>
> 👍 Like   💬 Comment

Holly's former student Erin posted on Holly's Facebook page.

Cynthia e-mailed:
Greg,

I just wanted to thank you for calling today. To say you have a lot on your plate right now is the understatement of the century. You are doing an amazing job in managing everything and everybody, given the terrifying nature of this all. I couldn't do what you are doing. Please know that we will all do the best on our end to relay info to one another and do whatever else we can to lighten the load just a little bit for you. Please reach out if you have any kind of need, no matter how stupid or small it is. Getting on a train to Long Island to bring you a sandwich, cutting and pasting names into an e-mail, whatever the task might be, I'm happy to do it.

Holly is very, very lucky to have such an amazing person at her side right now. You feel confident in the hands of the head surgeon, and I feel confident with Holly in your hands. Praying that surgery goes well…

From: Payan, Gregory
Sent: Wednesday, April 23, 2014, 9:43 p.m.
Subject: Holly Update Wednesday eve

All:

Again, a reminder to reply just to me and not to all. If someone should be on this list, please forward. My admin skills are sorely lacking as this list grows. Thanks.

Once more, thanks for the continued words of support. They mean the world. Holly has yet to hear all your beautiful words. I assure you she will when the time is right. In advance, please forgive grammar and typos, as sleep is elusive these days, and I am on fumes. I cannot speak, much less write, although I owe to all our cherished friends as much time as I can muster. I am eternally grateful to you all.

Today, unfortunately, can best be summed up as one step forward, two steps back. Holly is still strong and resting peacefully as I write this, but we did not have the result we had hoped for today. I will start with the bad and try to end positively.

The day started well, and the doctors felt good about accessing the aneurysm through the coil procedure. The coil basically goes into an artery in her groin and up to the base of her skull to get rid of the aneurysm…modern medicine. Wow. Everything went great until they were just about to access the aneurysm. Basically, the artery began to tear, so they aborted the procedure immediately. They sealed off the artery, and she's at no risk, as a result. She has another artery to the brain—actually 10 percent to 15 percent of the population has only one artery, but like most of the population, she has two. The aborted procedure is disheartening, but it caused her no harm that we can see. Her vitals are great, and she went in and out of anesthesia great. Her lungs and heart are solid. The doctors are confident she is ready for another, more invasive surgery tomorrow. Because of the increased sedation after the procedure, Holly spent most of the day resting very quietly, and we just held her hand or leg.

As a result of the failed coil procedure, they must go in through her skull tomorrow to access the aneurysm. The coil procedure is not possible through the other artery, for if something happened to the other artery, she would die. As I tried to convey yesterday, the aneurysm is rare, and it's in a terrible spot filled with neurological land mines. The doctor who will be performing the surgery has done thousands of aneurysm surgeries but only forty to fifty on this type of aneurysm. He is smart, experienced, and confident, but he is very honest in his assessment of the procedure and the difficulties involved. That said, if I could describe him, he's got thirty years of experience, and he's blunt in talking about the dangers, but he has an "I've got this covered" type of demeanor. Sharley and I are very pleased that he will be the one who holds Holly's future in his hands. We are hopeful but scared to death.

She is scheduled for an early morning surgery. I promise another e-mail at day's end tomorrow. Sooner, if I can manage. If there are delays, know that there are a lot of moving parts. If you do not hear from me, use the extra time to send good thoughts and prayers. Tomorrow will be brutal. There is a lot riding on the hands of a capable surgeon, and this surgery is not a sure thing. The worst is a possibility, a real one. Every ounce of my being hopes that I will correspond with you all with the best of news tomorrow eve.

Now that I have shared the bad of today and what is planned for tomorrow, I will share the good. Our Holly is remarkable. I got to the hospital this morn, and she was wide awake. I was greeted with a smile, and she asked for her pen and pad. We went back and forth for a few minutes as I gave her some info about things. Sadly, she was very scared when I told her why she was in the hospital again. (The nurse said I could, as she continues to forget.) Her brain is her most prized possession. She knows what an aneurysm means, and it was hard to convince her that her brain function right now is remarkable. She's scared to lose 1 percent of her brain, and she knows the perils of what happened to her.

The fact that we had this exchange basically forty-eight hours after she was unresponsive is nothing short of remarkable. If we get through tomorrow unscathed, with a perfect surgery, there is little doubt in my mind that she will get back to being the Holly we know and love: funny and brilliant and, yes, teasing me for not reading enough novels.

I want you all to be positive and thinking of her whenever you can tomorrow. She will need every last bit of good thoughts and prayers this community can extend in a spare moment—prayers of overwhelming love for her at all times, for strength for me and her family, for a surgeon's steady hand, and in the end, for many, many more years where we can share her company and bright eyes and laughter.

As with yesterday's update, thanks for all of the offers of visits, cards, flowers, etc. I will tell you all when the time is right, and that time is not now.

I thank you all from the bottom of my heart, as does Holly's sister, Sharley. I hope to be talking to you all tomorrow eve via this forum with the best of news.

Kerry e-mailed:
Greg,

I just happened to be online and am glad I am. I am relieved to hear from you with this news. Thank you again for taking the time to think of all of us in the midst of all of this. Clearly, Holly is a fighter and a survivor—with a wicked sense of humor. Love that, and I haven't even met her yet! I have seen that spirit before in my little girl, who has overcome a ton of tough days in her young years, including open-heart surgery. Those tough days are stories she and I share now, and I have faith that you and Holly will continue to make and share stories, this one in particular. Keep the faith. I will too, and I am sending you nothing but good vibes for a positive outcome tomorrow. The doctor sounds perfect. Am so glad he is there for Holly, you, and Sharley. I am saying a prayer every hour on the hour for all that you mentioned. Please know I am thinking of you. You and Holly are in my prayers.

Tanya e-mailed:
Dear Greg,

I'm so grateful that you are offering us this information and positivity and grace in the midst of what I know is your own personal dismay and reality. My husband had a small stroke in what was described by our neurologist as a "high-traffic area" ten years ago. It's not the same kind of scenario as you are describing but similar fear and unknowing. These years later, my husband still conducts his own financial-planning business; I serve Drew as the chaplain; and our kids, who were then fourteen (daughter) and eleven (twin daughter and son), are well-adjusted and have graduated college and are working. I believe deeply that Holly will recover and that you together will find your way forward. I pray for grace on this journey. I'm glad to know however Drew or I specifically can be of support. Peace and blessings.

Holly and I had been together for many years. As I mentioned earlier, Holly had married her high school sweetheart. It was a happy marriage that ended tragically when he died of liver cancer. She maintained a strong relationship with her in-laws for many years after his death and spoke of them in the most wonderful of terms. Despite the many years Holly and I had been together, I never had met her in-laws. It had always bothered me. While it had come up many times in our relationship, Holly always would find a reason for me not to meet them as we traveled in Texas: She did not have time to call them... They were likely busy. Standard excuses not grounded in reality, but I accepted them respectfully, because Holly clearly did not want this meeting to happen.

A few times I did press Holly about it, expressing my desire to meet them. Eventually, Holly acknowledged she just felt the meeting would be awkward. Her in-laws were evangelical Christians who were very religious and living in a conservative state. I was a lapsed Catholic who had grown up in Queens, New York. She was nervous the meeting would be uncomfortable and that we would not "connect." She thought it safer for us not to meet, rather than for people who all shared a common bond in their love for her to have absolutely nothing else in common and come away from their meeting sad and/or disappointed. It bothered me for years that she would prefer we never meet, but I acquiesced.

Now, as Holly was readying for her next surgery, I felt this incredible urge to speak with her late husband's parents, though I never had spoken with them before. Once it was clear that Holly was going to undergo her dangerous craniotomy and could not stop me from speaking with them, I asked Sharley to get me their phone number, which she did.

What did I want to say? I can't really remember. My main goal was to let them know that since I'd been with Holly, she had been loved with every ounce of my being. I was never there to replace their son, who Holly always honored, but I wanted to let them know I had done the best I could since being with Holly and that she was happy, was treated well, and loved our time together. And if she did not make it through the surgery, I wanted them to know she had lived every minute since their son had died. She had lived a life that honored him through her actions and her words. And she had done it with me by her side, encouraging her every step of the way.

Please Stay

    I called Holly's in-laws the night before her craniotomy and spoke with them for about half an hour from a quiet area near the elevator bank at the hospital. I sat on a wide windowsill, as it was quieter and actually a bit more private than the ICU waiting room. When I introduced myself, they were seemingly expecting my call, so Sharley likely had tipped them off. They put me on speakerphone so I could speak to them both at once. I never had the faith of a strong believer in God, but I drew great strength from my conversation with them. They were beautiful people. While not sharing their strong belief in God, I felt worlds better having spoken with them. Their faith that Holly would make it through the surgery and return to her former self gave me strength. I cannot explain how, but it did. I was so grateful for that call. I also hung up the phone a little angry at Holly that she had not let me share time with them for the last ten-plus years. There are few people I have ever come across with such pure hearts, who are believers that all would, in fact, be OK. On that night, their belief gave me strength. I would need every bit of it to help me through tomorrow.

Demy e-mailed:
Hi Greg,

    Thank you so much for taking the time to write us updates and to deal with our calls, texts, etc. Cynthia filled me in today, and I can tell you (as you can imagine, I hope) that not a moment passes without me thinking of our wonderful, marvelous, and sweet Holly. I love the story where she teased you—her spirit is so strong, and she is a fighter! She is in my thoughts and prayers all the time, and when I pause for a second, I see her beautiful smile, and I think of our last time together at the pub, talking about the Oscars and blogs…I had to teach today (that was so hard, especially as I could think of all the talks I have had with Holly about teaching), and she was in my thoughts the whole time. I ended up letting my students out forty-five minutes early—all I could think of was what was happening with Holly. That is way more important at this point. (Students were thrilled, of course.) I am hoping tomorrow will bring us all the results we want and are praying for: Holly being a step closer to getting this aneurysm. I will be hopeful…Thanks for *your* encouragement and for keeping us all connected. I will pray hard and hope for the best because this has to be our only possible outcome.

Nancy e-mailed:
Greg,
Your updates are remarkable and a welcome gift for those of us who are far away. Thank you, thank you, thank you. My prayers are steady, and my love and positive thoughts and strength are all on full blast and pointed in Holly's direction. I'm holding you and Sharley in my heart at all times. I find myself saying aloud, "Come on, Holly! You got this," about twice an hour. I realize that people around me must think I'm nuts, but I care not. It makes me feel like the words and will can make it to her faster all the way from California.

I will be thinking of all of you constantly tomorrow. I wish there was more I could do. Hang in there. She's got this.

Inge e-mailed:
Dear Holly,
Please don't be mad at me, but I did not light a candle for you in Sacre Coeur Basilica yesterday like I promised. I walked into the church and thought, Hmmmm, this isn't Holly. I need to find something better.

So I walked around the corner to the very old church of Saint Pierre, which has actually been around since the eleventh century, whereas the basilica dates to the late nineteenth. Imagine, for thousands of years people have been going to Saint Pierre with hearts bursting with hopes and fears to ask their god for whatever. That's what I did for you yesterday and again today, both times in the early morning before any tourists were around. And from up there, you have a wonderful view of all of Paris, of course. A sprawling city where people live and love and make mistakes and sometimes get it right and all the rest of it. And above it all, a candle burns just for you in the old Saint Pierre church.

Holly, I'll take you and Greg there when next you are in Paris. In Saint Pierre, I have a favorite stained-glass window. It shows the walking on the water, and all you see are wavy blue lines that represent water and bare footprints. I love it! Just think, if a man can walk on water, what can a woman do? Especially a strong, smart one like yourself. And from what I hear, you've been cracking jokes and flirting with your nurse, which is nothing short of miraculous, as far as I'm concerned. I hope Greg isn't jealous.

Anyway, I am thinking and praying for you and sending loads and loads of amour to you and Greg.

As Holly pursued her PhD, she sometimes reminded me that she was not supposed to be here—"here" being an academic studying and learning with renowned scholars in her field, writing a dissertation that likely would be published as a book upon completion. "I'm just the daughter of an auto mechanic," she would say. It was her way of reiterating that her academic success was unlikely, and it shouldn't have happened, based on her background in suburban Texas. Maybe this story held wisdom for what she was about to endure the next morning. She had been a long shot to make it through her initial bleed. She was also going to be a long shot to get through the surgery with a good outcome. Maybe the "daughter of an auto mechanic" was here to defy odds. The "daughter of an auto mechanic" was fierce though and had Hillgardner blood in her. That meant she was her father's daughter, and he was as strong as they come. Maybe she'd defy the odds once more, I kept telling myself as I eventually drifted off to some fitful sleep that night.

DAY 4—THE CRANIOTOMY
April 24, 2014

IN THE PREDAWN HOURS BEFORE *Holly's craniotomy, Sharley and I were struck with a feeling of helplessness. A tragic result was a distinct possibility. Another possibility was that Holly could come out of the surgery with cognitive deficits. Most would argue that this was more likely than not, in spite of her brain functioning pretty well after the bleed. This surgery involved sawing into her skull and trying to access an aneurysm in a bad spot, inches from where they entered, while trying not to touch or affect anything along the way. An inch is a small measurement in the real world, but inside a brain, it's a frighteningly long distance when you consider the brain is made of more than 100 billion neurons that communicate through billions more connections that control our bodies and lives. Holly's aneurysm needed to be accessed on her basilar artery, which is located at the base of the skull—much too long a distance from the surgery's entry point for my comfort. Her surgeon would have to navigate a neurological minefield to access it without touching anything vital.*

Before they took her to the operating room, I talked to the surgeon. With watery eyes, I said, "I know how Holly wants to live life. If something goes drastically wrong, she does not want to live in a compromised state."

He gave me a penetrating look. "We're not there yet," he said. "I feel good." He projected a calm spirit and seemed to think it was possible to pull this off, in spite of the odds against it.

Holly would be in the operating room for hours, so Sharley and I wrote her a note. We did this not knowing whether she'd come out or what condition she'd be in if she did. We needed something, a part of us, even words on paper, to be with her. We taped the note under her bed (the same one she'd be on during her surgery) and told her we loved her, and then it was time. She was wheeled off for surgery, and we went to the waiting room.

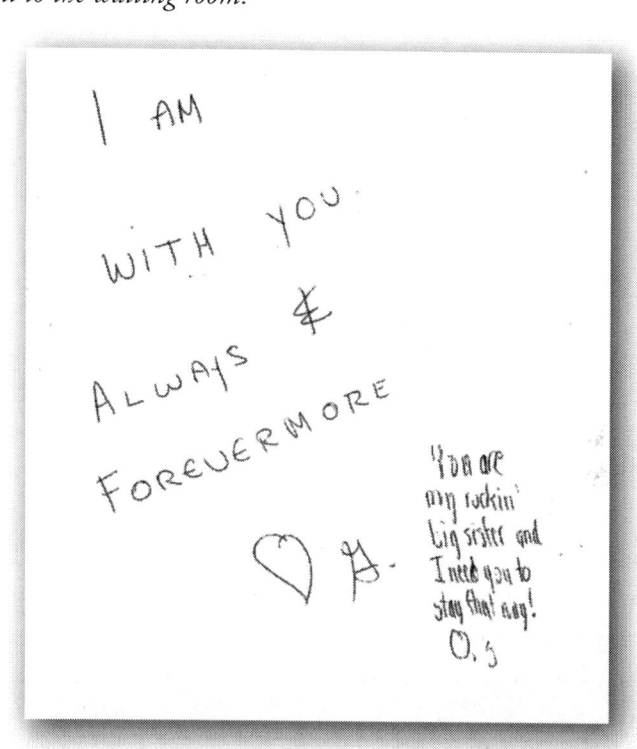

> I AM WITH YOU & ALWAYS & FOREVERMORE
>
> ♡ A.
>
> You are my rockin' big sister and I need you to stay that way!
>
> O, J

I wrote this at a moment's notice, fearing more than anything else that Holly would feel alone and scared in the surgery.

The notes continued to come as I searched for a way to pass the time during one of the longest days of my life.

—

Danielle e-mailed:
My dearest Greg,
    I know that my words cannot provide adequate comfort to you while your dear, sweet Holly is going through these difficult procedures. I know that having her home again with you is your only focus. Please know that you and

she have been in my constant thoughts since Denise alerted me. I pray that today yields good news.

Greg, I know and care about you exactly the same as when we were young. There is something about becoming childhood friends that leaves an indelible mark that remains even though we are not able to see each other often. I hope you know that you have friends everywhere who wish to support you and Holly in any way we can.

I will be thinking of Holly, her sister and family, and you throughout the day. I will be anxiously awaiting news on her condition.

I replied to Danielle:

Thanks, Danielle. Holly is in surgery right now, and this helps me pass the time. I can say that as years go by and I follow your travels on Facebook, I am oft reminded of Holly when I see your pix. I would imagine that you are quite similar—fiercely independent and beautiful and loving to travel, even alone. That is how I met Holly ten years ago on a beach in Mexico as we both traveled alone. Ten years of memories later brings us to a really bad place this week. I am hopeful but oh so scared. Thanks for the notes and prayers. Keep them coming.

Danielle responded:

I certainly will keep the prayers coming, Greg; the two of you have not ever been far from my thoughts these last couple days. I know Holly through your pictures, so I know how beautiful she is. Somehow, a bit of our personalities also come through our pictures. I am not quite sure how that happens, but I like to think that I have a sense of who Holly is. Also, knowing you, I know that she must be a wonderful person. As we get older (I am not quite sure how that happened to us, Greg!), I have learned two things: 1) People are the whole thing. 2) We are not as in control as we think we are, so adaptability may be our most important quality. This is just too much to be happening to someone so dear; it is difficult to even comprehend. I know that you are scared, but this is so completely beyond your control, so try to just keep looking forward to the next step, if you can. However, in the meantime, while you are waiting in the waiting room, try to think of that Mexican beach with Holly! Nice warm sun…beautiful water…Holly….:)

Wanda e-mailed:
Greg,

Sending much love, healing light, blessings, heavenly protection, strength, peace, calm, and endurance. We are all pulling for you and Holly…You're doing really well…You have divine support surrounding and protecting you…as does Holly.

Breathe deep.

Love to you, my friend.

God is with you…

Marjorie e-mailed:
Greg,

I went out to the beach yesterday to say a prayer for Holly. The waves were unsurfable, and I thought it was the ocean's way of saying, "We're mad about Holly." :)

I made a wish for you all and threw it into the sea. I am thinking of her night and day and know I will hear good news later.

She's amazing, as are you!

Kara e-mailed:
Hi Greg,

I am sending prayers and love throughout the day and night your and Holly's way. I am Holly's old friend (first yoga teacher—yes, the journey of Holly's yoga started with our little group in Arlington, and the student became the master!) from Texas. I visited Holly and met you in New York a few years ago—Holly and I went to Greece together a few years back as well.

I remember when Holly first told me about you. She was absolutely smitten when she met you. She told me stories about leaving her couch on the sidewalk when she moved to New York—only to have it snapped up minutes later—while moving into that cool first apartment. But she said it was all worth it because of you. Couch or no couch.

I know she must always keep you on your toes, and you must be an amazing person to keep her on her toes. So thank you for being her soul mate and holding her hand through this. Please give Shar a hug for me.

To Holly when she is ready:

To my amazing friend and inspiration—my inspiration to be fearless and full of light and love. I love you so much and can't wait to see you soon. Let the doctors help heal you, but your fierce independence will get you through this. I am bringing my Birkenstocks to walk around Queens with you as soon as you're ready. All my love.

1:49 p.m.
HH texted:
Greg, how was the surgery?
Let me know if you have time, but only if you have time.

I replied:
Still in surgery
No updates
Waiting
Will give you a quick call momentarily.
I'd like to hear your voice.
My family is here, but I need to hear
from one of Holly's Texas friends.

―⁓―

I likely spent an hour talking in my head to Holly during her surgery that day. I had put her favorite ring (the rocksy-proxy ring) on a chain and wore it around my neck. During her surgery, I would touch the ring and whisper repeatedly, as if it were a mantra, "I am with you. Don't be scared."

Sharley, on the other hand, would walk by the operating room. From the hallway, you could see a closed-circuit feed from every operating room where a surgery was happening. It was not nearly close enough to see what was happening—it was more like bad security video from a convenience store—but Shar kept trying to figure out which feed was Holly's.

I was instructed not to watch the clock during the surgery, although I couldn't help but do so. My assumption is that doctors do not want loved ones thinking that if a surgery takes longer than expected, things are going poorly. I did a lot of pacing and talking to my family and Sharley. Tommy, one of my closest friends, who works at a hospital, came by for a few hours to wait with me as well. I remember listening to a lot of music, as I could not even begin to focus on reading. At one point, I played a song Holly and I had always said we'd play at our wedding. That song was "The Beatitudes" by the Kronos Quartet. I remember asking my mother to listen to it with me; I gave her an earbud and held her hand as we said a silent prayer.

Holly's surgery lasted a bit over six hours, but I remember being in the waiting room for about eight, considering the surgery prep time and such. The first four or five hours, I wandered a bit and tried to eat. After that, I couldn't help but stare at the door, waiting for the surgeon to come out with an update. Eventually, long after I expected him to, Holly's doctor came out of the door in his blue scrubs and walked immediately toward me. He smelled as if he had just worked out. The pressure and tension of being in charge of leading a team through more than six hours of neurosurgery is something I will never comprehend.

My first thought, before he spoke, was that whatever had gone on in the operating room likely had been a struggle. He confirmed that quickly. The surgery was successful—but not before the aneurysm reruptured as he tried to clip it. He was not happy. He stated quite directly that any time there are complications during brain surgery, it's bad. He did say that if there was something to draw hope from, it was that his team had controlled the situation. And even when the aneurysm reruptured, Holly's vital signs had remained steady. He drew a straight line in the air with his hand to illustrate that there were no dips in her breathing, blood pressure, or other vital signs. "Solid as a rock," he said.

Holly was stable, but complications may not be noticeable until she regained consciousness. "Now we wait," he said.

My parents, Tommy, Sharley, and I went up to the ICU waiting room, where I sobbed into my cry towel, which was still on my shoulder, for a minute or two, maybe because the surgery did not go perfectly or maybe because I just needed an emotional release. Maybe I cried for an uncertain future or for all I thought we would become and potentially never would be after everything that had happened.

Sharley tried to emphasize that everything looked good. The aneurysm was gone, clipped, and we did not have to worry about it anymore. The rest of the family felt the same way. Maybe I did, too, but at that point, I was just spent. I had nothing left.

Holly was transferred back to her ICU room, and I was able to say good night to her, though she was not conscious. I went back to my parents' home to try to calm down. Sharley stayed at the hospital for a few more hours.

―◦―

This is the report about Holly's craniotomy and the successful clipping of the aneurysm. While there is a lot of medical jargon, there are also times during the report when the lack of clinical terminology stands out—particularly when her surgeon notes at the end of a long, difficult surgery with complications that, once done, "Everything looked good."

NORTH SHORE UNIVERSITY HOSPITAL

PATIENT: Hillgardner, Holly
DATE OF OPERATION: 04/24/2014
ENCOUNTER #: 500007441586

OPERATIVE REPORT
DOB: 07/01/1974
PREOPERATIVE DIAGNOSIS: Basilar artery apex aneurysm
POSTOPERATIVE DIAGNOSIS: Basilar artery apex aneurysm

NATURE OF OPERATION: Under SSEP, EEG and motor-evoked potential monitoring, right-sided pterional craniotomy with craniorbital zygomatic approach and micro dissection, clipping of basilar artery aneurysm, and microvascular Doppler of posterior circular Willis vessels.

PROCEDURE: The patient was brought into the operating room and placed under general endotracheal anesthesia. Venous, arterial, and Foley lines were set, and the patient was placed in the three-pin head holder in the standard position for a right-sided craniotomy. SSEP and EEG potential leads were placed on the patient's head in addition to motor-evoked potential leads and baseline potentials were obtained and they stayed constant throughout the entirety of the operation. A standard aneurysm incision was outlined and it was opened with a #10 blade. Raney clamps and Danoy clamps were applied bilaterally and the scalp flap was reflected back and held in place with Yasargil scalp hooks. The temporalis muscle was freed from its bed and held posteriorly in the standard fashion with Yasargil scalp hooks. A standard four burr holes were then made with the Midas rex drill, and a standard pterional craniotomy was harvested. The scalp flap was further dissected anteriorly and with the use of a sagittal saw, a standard cranial orbital zygomatic ostectomy was made, and this was lifted out in two pieces without injury to any underlying tissue, specifically, the periorbita. These bone plates were safe for later use, and at the end of the operation, were plated back into position. At this point, we had a white dural exposure, and the zygoma and the orbital rim and roof had been resected. Holes were drilled in the calgarium, and the dura was tacked up with 4-0 silk sutures, and absolute epidural hemostasis was obtained. The dura was opened in a curvilinear fashion and flapped up toward the sphenoid wing, and the surface of the brain showed evidence of recent subarachnoid hemorrhage with orange staining. The rest of the operation was performed under the Zeiss operating microscope.

Under the operating microscope, the sylvian fissure was widely opened from lateral to medial, and the arachnoidal adhesions between the optic nerve and the frontal lobe were taken down. Once this was done, we identified the carotid artery, the anterior choroidal artery, and the posterior communicating artery. There was an extremely small optical carotid triangle, so it became apparent immediately that the dissection down into the interpeduncular cistern would be performed lateral to the internal carotid artery. A gentle frontal retractor was left in place, and a deep temporal retractor was used to access this zone. We followed the posterior communicating artery under high magnification until we were able to see the junction of the posterior communicating artery with the P2 segment. We never retracted the carotid artery with a retractor, and the temporal retraction and the angulation of the microscope coupled with the COZ approach gave us an excellent view into this region. We eventually identified the P1 segment on the right side, and this led us to the basilar apex. This was an extremely tedious, difficult dissection, and it was a very deep exposure with limited mobility. The posterior clinoid process somewhat obscured the proximal basilar artery as the area of the superior cerebellar on the right and the left and both P1 takeoffs had a bulbous appearance, and this was consistent with what was seen on the angiogram.

Eventually, we were able to dissect the ipsilateral P1 segment from the aneurysm neck, and by looking across the basilar artery were able to see some more vertically oriented contralateral P1 segment. A 15-mm straight titanium Yasargil clip was placed cleanly across the neck of the aneurysm at this point without temporary arterial occlusion, and I was satisfied the aneurysm had been occluded. There was no change in the evoked potentials or the vital signs. Under extremely high magnification, I inspected the clip, and it appeared to pinch approximately 40 percent to 50 percent of the contralateral proximal P1 segment. With the clip remover, I opened the clip to back it off ever so slightly, and there was an intraoperative rupture at this point. This was a difficult intraoperative rupture to control, and eventually I was able to see the point of bleeding at the basilar apex, and the same clip was put into position slightly deeper, and the bleeding stopped. At this point, I suspected that the P1 segment was within the clip, and further dissection did show that the P1 segment was within the clip. The aneurysm was completely clipped. Microvascular Doppler was then performed on the Circle of Willis vessels. There was an excellent signal from the right-sided P1 and superior cerebella and the basilar, and there was a weaker but present signal from the P1 segment on the left side. I attempted to back off the clip again, but there was bleeding from the aneurysm, so eventually the clip was left in position, and I was counting on collateral flow through the large-caliber left-sided posterior communicating artery. At this point, I was confident a complete clipping had been achieved. Despite the intraoperative rupture, everything looked good. The brain was relaxed and pulsatile, and the retractors were removed from the brain, and absolute hemostasis was achieved. Once this was done, the dura was reconstituted with 4–0 silk sutures and absolute epidural hemostasis was achieved. The craniotomy was plated back into position with standard plates, and the COZ construct was reconstructed with plates. The temporalis muscle was reconstituted with 3–0 Vicryl sutures, and the scalp was closed with 3–0 Vicryl for galea and staples for skin. Prior to this, a Jackson-Pratt drain was laid into position in the subglaeal compartment. A dry sterile dressing was applied. The patient was taken out of the three-pin head holder and brought out immediately for a CT scan, which showed standard postoperative changes, and she was brought to the neurosurgical intensive care unit in stable condition.

FINAL DIAGNOSIS: Ruptured basilar artery apex aneurysm
PROCEDURE: Right-sided craniotomy with COZ approach and clipping of basilar apex aneurysm.

From:	Payan, Gregory
Sent:	Thursday, April 24, 2014, 6:53 p.m.
Subject:	Holly Update Thursday

All:

First and foremost, Holly made it through the surgery. Her vitals are stable. This, alone, is cause for some celebration. When I arrived at the hospital, I did not know if she'd be with us at day's end. I cannot convey enough how difficult and dangerous this surgery was. It was a deep, small aneurysm that was very hard to get to. It is now gone. But she is far from out of the woods yet.

The surgery took over six hours. When the surgeon was clipping the aneurysm, it reruptured and bled again. The bleeding eventually was controlled, and the clip was put in place. The doctor feels confident about the clip. It is rock-solid and not moving. The aneurysm will no longer be an issue. The bad side is that there was significant bleeding during the surgery. Any complication is not a good thing, and this was a significant complication. He ordered an immediate CT scan to see if anything bad showed up. Nothing did, and he emphasized that her vitals stayed rock-solid throughout the entire process. This, too, is great, but his optimism is guarded at best.

I am still frightened beyond words. I should, however, emphasize that Sharley, Holly's sister, is positive. Her view is that Holly's vitals are great, the CT scan is clean, and the aneurysm is gone. We can deal with the rest.

The doctor says he is neither positive nor negative. The next twelve to seventy-two hours will mean a lot, he feels. He is a world-class neurosurgeon, and he emphasized that he did not want to do the surgery (hoping the initial "coiling" would work, because installing the clip in the area of Holly's aneurysm would be difficult and invasive) and that there were complications, so he does not feel good about things. That said, her vitals and CT scan are clean. There is no reason to believe that she came out of it badly, but he needs twenty-four hours to feel better about it.

Holly will be under constant care from her army of doctors and nurses for the next twenty-four hours. She will be getting the best of care. She is strong and fierce and resilient. Her miraculous recovery from Monday proved that, but our girl has had a rough week. What she has endured this week is Herculean. If her condition and all neurological signs are good for the next twenty-four hours, there will be a collective exhale. Seventy-two hours…even better. She will still have to worry about complications, infections, and vasospasms (a sudden constriction of the blood vessels that could lead to a stroke), but a significant hurdle will have been cleared. This process will take three weeks before there is even a thought of her being discharged. It's a marathon, not a sprint.

Again, the words of support continue to give me strength, but I ask that you please not forget Holly's sister, Sharley. If you know her, send her a note too. If you don't know her, still send her a note. Her spirit this week has been remarkable and really puts me to shame. She is optimistic and smiling and has made this ordeal better for me—and more important, better for Holly.

Before you even think about sending me a note, I beg you to please tell Sharley how wonderful she is and how much you love and care about Holly. She deserves it so very much.

I am sorry this isn't the fairy tale we'd hoped for as I sign off this evening. It still has that possibility, but we're not there yet. Not even close. I am very fond of the lead character in this story, though, and I think we all echo the thought that few people are more prepared for this fight than Holly is.

Please keep the love and prayers on overdrive. There's a beautiful and special woman in Manhasset that this world needs who is in desperate need of the best you can offer over the next few weeks.

Thank you all for the love and support.

Keely e-mailed:
Greg,

I know the road will be long, but me and a lot of other people are on it with y'all every step of the way. Even though it may feel like we aren't b/c of the geographical distance. Just say the word, and I will be on a plane. But I know probably everyone feels that way, but I really can do it. I've got nothing keeping me in Austin.

Holly will be able to do anything required for recovery, if anyone can. She made it through today, so now on to the next twelve to seventy-two hours, then the next week and week and week.

OK, hang in there. You are doing great. Again, let me know anything I can do or send.

Kevin e-mailed:
Greg,

You are stronger than most men.

Holly is in my thoughts and prayers. Hoping for all good news in the upcoming hours/days. We'll all be laughing over drinks soon enough again.

<u>**7:19 p.m.**</u>
I texted Shar:
How is our girl doing?

Shar replied:
She's taking it easy.
Starting to stir a little in response to her name,
but meds still wearing off.
They said she just needs more time.
All vitals are good.

I texted:
Thank you. Xoxoxo. You're the best.

Shar replied:
I know! Lol
I keep getting Facebook private messages
from people saying they just heard from you.
I sent you home for some downtime!

I texted:
I sent an update on Holly and reminded them
to drop you a note for how spectacular you are.
No reason I should get all the nice notes.

Sam e-mailed:
Greg,

Thanks so much for what must be a fairly excruciating set of e-mails to write. It sounds like today brought at least a kernel of hope. I just want you to know that it's wonderful to see your love for Holly and to know that you are there with her. On behalf of the many who worry from afar, I'm glad Holly has you there. And I'm profoundly grateful for your taking the time to send these updates.

When the time is appropriate, please tell Holly that I've got a bunch of folks at our church here in North Carolina praying for her and that they have been checking with me to see how she's doing. She hasn't met any of them, but they're wonderful people, and their prayers are joining the chorus you've been conducting this week.

John e-mailed:
Greg,

This is JG, and we have met several times when you were in West Virginia. If I remember correctly, it was the first time you had ever seen a hummingbird, which I still sort of chuckle about.

At any rate, I was hoping you would add me to your e-mail list so that I can keep getting updates. I made a brief post or two on my website asking my readers to keep her in their thoughts (it's a very caring community), and I received a couple of e-mails from people in New York City who are willing to do anything you need to help.

When I was at the post office today, I told the postmaster to hold Holly's mail, and I believe my father is going to be picking up her car from the airport tomorrow, so she is not being charged out the wazoo.

At any rate, I just want you to know that the two of you are in our thoughts, and if there is anything I can do, please let me know. I check this e-mail compulsively.

Aileen e-mailed:
Dearest Greg,

I am so relieved and happy to hear that Holly made it out of surgery, that her vitals are strong, and that her CT scan is clear. This is all good news. I have been with you all day, praying, thinking of you both, and looking forward to a time when we can all get together for a good meal and put this bad memory behind us. That day will come. I am sure of it.

For now, please remember that you and Holly have a lot of love surrounding you and lifting you up. Try to take things day by day, hour by hour, if necessary, and try not let yourself worry about the "what ifs" too much. I know how incredibly hard that will be. You got good news today, and though the days ahead will be extremely rough and trying, you both will get through this. Please remember that it is the doctor's job to be cautious and guarded. It is, I believe, the sign of a good doctor. Tomorrow will be a new day, and hopefully, Holly will begin quickly to show signs of improvement.

You are one of my very closest friends, Greg, and it pains me terribly that you and Holly are suffering. I wish I could be there with you to help you through this. I continue to think about you both and will pray every day for her quick recovery.

Tanya e-mailed:
Dear Greg,

I have just sent Sharley a message on behalf of the Drew Theological School community, but I want to continually thank you for keeping us apprised of Holly's condition and being vulnerable in your own expression of anxiety, fear, and waiting.

We are so glad to hear that Holly came through this morning's surgery with such strength. We did stop our chapel service this morning to pray with you and Holly and Holly's family, knowing she was in the midst of the procedure. We sent as much positive resurrection energy as we could muster to you all and hope that it was felt. Please know that we are here, a steady and present community, ready to help, but knowing now that our best help is to be communicating our prayers to you and Holly.

Maura e-mailed:
Hi Greg,

I'm so glad I'm able to access my work e-mail at home. When I saw that you said Holly made it through the surgery, I clapped my hands. I have been thinking of her all day and continue to pray for her. I sent a note to her sister, as you requested.

Continued prayers for you and Sharley as well for strength and fortitude during such a difficult time.

Austin e-mailed:
Dear Holly,

I spoke with God about you this morning. It didn't take me long to know that everything I told the Lord was meant for you, too.

I told the Lord that I hope for love and grace to bear you up and that in this time you would know mercy and you would know peace. I told the Lord that you have reflected and borne so much hope and encouragement to me and a thousand others, and I prayed that now you would somehow receive that back in this time when you need it most.

I thanked the Lord for you and for the moment you came into my life. I thought about each year at Arlington High. English. Creative Writing. Lit Mag. I thought about how I learned from you and how I became a better person by you. I never found out how it was for you at home in that time. What I saw, though, was a brilliant, strong woman showing people how to broaden their minds and do things that are great, even as other things weren't so great at all.

I think it worked. I'm pretty sure your students went on to do great things. Thanks to you.

I told God all of this, and you gotta know there were tears in my eyes then, and there are tears in my eyes now.

You're going to be there, though, Holly. When I get poems and essays published. When I sell my first novel. Anytime I find the right word for the right occasion, your legacy is there—you know that, right? And dammit, I want to show them to you. I want you to have the proof of your greatness as a teacher in your hands. I want you to be very old and thinking, Wow, I made a lot of great things happen. I want you to rest content, knowing you made the most and the best of your days.

So I said that, too, to God, and I realized it's kinda selfish (oh bloody well), but more importantly, I realized you should be able to rest in that right now. You have lived and given and experienced so much, and you are loved, and you are known, and you have made an impact.

Take this letter as a hug if I do not get to see you soon. If you do not hear the words from my voice, let this then stand to say, thank you, Holly Hillgardner, for being a teacher, a mentor, and a friend.

You'll be with us always, O Captain! My captain! And I pray to see you and thank you face-to-face many times yet.

Emily e-mailed:
Greg,

I will e-mail Sharley to let her know she's amazing, but *you* are amazing too, and I am blown away at your fortitude these last few days. I hope you get the chance to rest to gear up for the rest of the week. I am so relieved that the surgery is over and that she is through it.

Holly will get through anything, no matter what, even if it's rehab or whatever she needs. She'll get through it, and I really believe and hope with all my heart that she will be the Holly we know and love. Please take care of yourself as much as possible right now. Thank you for your beautiful updates. I am thinking of you and Holly and Sharley every second.

So many people love Holly; I had no idea how many friends she had. She was always just *my* friend. I'm happy to share her with everyone when she is better.

11:03 p.m.
I texted Shar:
Any idea a good time to go tomorrow?
I might be asleep soon.
Can you call the nurse station and text me?
a basic update or call if I need to know something?
The phone is by my side.

Shar replied:
Go to bed.
I will probably still be here.
No update, she is still very sleepy.
I say 8:00 a.m.
Nothing new to change that plan.

I texted:
OK.
Thanks so much.
See you then.

Shar replied:
You may be on your own in a.m. for a bit.
Depends on how late I stay.
I am singing and playing music for her!
See you. Xoxo

I texted:
Tell her nurse he's awesome,
and make sure he reminds her whenever he can
that Greg and Shar love her
and will see her in morn—

Shar replied:
Already did!
Just leaving now.
She is still very sleepy,
but she opens her left eye a smidge,
and she is moving her legs well.
Arms some, not as much.
Very good news!

Lydia e-mailed:
Greg,

It isn't my usual response to situations like this, but from the beginning, I've felt confident that Holly is gonna come out of this, only more herself than ever. Holly's combination of mental, spiritual, and physical intelligence doesn't just testify to her love, strength, and passion for life; these are more than feelings and experiences. They are deep habits of mind/body integration that are working nonstop for her right now. Holly's life practices are so many neural pathways long used to lighting up in new ways, creatively unfolding, refusing refusals, pursuing alternatives, making connections, finding a way.

I think she is prepared for this.
I think she's got this.
I believe in Holly.

The night of Holly's craniotomy was one of my hardest. Holly had undergone invasive brain surgery. I did not know who she would be when she recovered and how this would affect her, me, or us. Nobody wants to be a long-term caregiver. It's something that's thrust upon you by circumstances. After she made it through this ordeal—or rather, if she made it through—would I become her caregiver?

In the first few days after Holly's rupture, I was forced to confront issues within myself that I had always tried to avoid. Holly and I had mutually decided not to have kids. She had her reasons, and I knew my personality was not conducive to parenting. It terrified me to think about having children and being unable to control their lives, their happiness. I knew I would want them never to experience loss or heartbreak or sickness. I would want to protect them from anything bad that can be experienced in the world. Now, with Holly sick and enduring pain, I was slowly losing my mind.

All I wanted to do was make it better. All I wanted to do was rewind events to the life we'd had before the rupture. All I wanted to do was eliminate her suffering. But I could not. My inability to do that would torture me in the coming weeks and months.

DAY 5 — RETURNING TO OUR APARTMENT WITHOUT HER
April 25, 2014

8:20 a.m.
I texted Shar:
Talked to doc.
All looks good.
Only slight issue is some slight abnormal electricity activity in brain,
which could lead to seizures.
All else good.
Responding to commands while still on heavy sedatives.

Shar replied:
OK!
We are coming over in a bit.
See you then.

I texted:
The mood is upbeat.

Shar replied:
How is your mood?

I texted:
Good.
Will be better if angiogram is performed and is clean.
It will show how tight the clip is and if it's leaking.
That is tentative for this morn.
Doc yesterday was real confident though,
so I'm praying it's just a formality.

Shar replied:
That's great.
So let's play "Brave" now and then later "Happy."

I texted:
Doing so now.

We played Sara Bareilles's song "Brave" repeatedly during Holly's stay in the ICU and in rehab, for obvious reasons. It also happened to be the same song she'd played to get herself psyched for her dissertation defense the previous year. Often we'd play it on the iPad in her room and sometimes through headphones. To this day, I cannot hear it without immediately being taken back to those days. In our desperate search for anything additional to bring us strength, that song helped.

Carol e-mailed:
Dear Greg and Sharley,
   I am not big on prayer, and words tend to fail me, but please know this: I truly believe Holly will be OK. She has to be…there can be no other outcome.

Holly made it through the surgery and was stable, but I could not yet comprehend what "stable" was. We did not know what she'd be like when she became aware of her surroundings and began to speak (if she could). We did not know what would be different postsurgery. I was full of questions: What would her personality be like? Would she maybe have a droopy eye? Would she have full use of her limbs? Would she have balance issues? How would her intelligence be affected? There were no answers to those questions. All of these were possibilities, according to the doctors, but only time would provide the answers.

There was also the fact that I just could not wrap my head around neurosurgery. Doctors had cut open her skin and peeled it back, sawed into her skull, and entered her brain for microsurgery. A clip had "sealed off" the aneurysm and restored normal blood flow into and around her brain. How does a layperson comprehend that? How was she to function next week or next month, much less for the next fifty years, with this tiny piece of titanium holding together her circulatory system—literally separating life from death? Would this clip prevent the inevitable? For how long? What would our life be like? Would anything be the same as it had been before?

"One day at a time" is the oft-repeated advice we all have heard when dealing with an intense crisis or challenging time in our lives, and that's exactly what it came down to. I would just focus on making it to tomorrow and figure the rest out later.

There was a collective exhale the day after the craniotomy. I checked on Holly in the morning. The medical team was running a myriad of tests, so Sharley and I took the opportunity to run back to my apartment for the first time since Holly had been wheeled out to the ambulance five days earlier. I needed clothes, as I would be staying at my parents' home awhile longer.

I was curious about how emotional I would be in the apartment where it all had happened. It felt like going back to a crime scene. The cup of coffee I had made for Holly on Monday morning sat on the counter untouched, a thin layer of mold atop it, along with her untouched breakfast. The bedroom, where she'd had the seizure, was in disarray—sheets half off the bed and some dirty clothing on the floor that had not made it to the hamper the night before.

Thankfully, I was OK as I surveyed the rooms. My brain was able to separate the terrifying medical incident from the memories of good times we'd had in the apartment. A part of me had worried I might not be able to separate the two. Sharley and I cleaned up and then packed some clothes for the week ahead. We also grabbed photos and the framed print that hung next to our bed to decorate Holly's room in the ICU. We had an hour or two free from the hospital, but Holly *was in a lot of pain, and we were anxious to return to make sure things were progressing and that her vitals would continue to improve and she'd soon regain consciousness.*

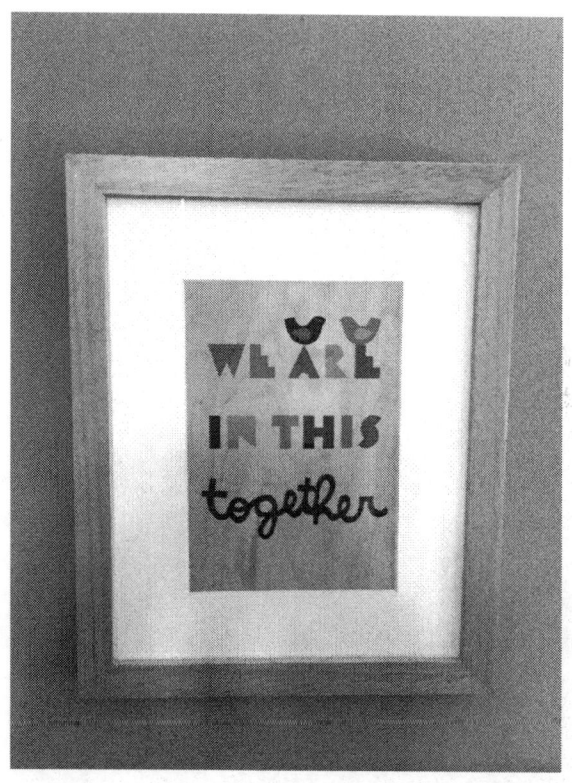

This print hung in Holly's room in the hospital and later in rehab.

Brian e-mailed:
Hope the night went well, and we are extremely happy that Holly got thru the surgery. She is crazy strong and will get thru this. Definitely feel free to call me if you need anything or just want some company. Take care, buddy.

I replied to Brian:
Can you keep Saturday eve open? If she stays stable, I may just need a night with you guys. Maybe watch a basketball game and have a few beers at my parents'. She's getting the best care here. Let's see how tomorrow shakes out. As you can imagine, I am wrecked.

Brian responded:
You got it. I got my nephew's communion at 1:30, but it'll be over by 5. Tell me when and where, and I'll be there.

I replied to Brian:
Float it to Charlie, Kieran, Elvis, and Alex too if they are available. Won't be a go until early or midafternoon based on her condition, but I think I can use it if Sharley can hang at the hospital for a bit. We've been doing shifts, and maybe I can swing the early on Saturday. Thanks.

Brian responded:
Done and done. Let me know your status whenever you get the chance on Saturday, and let me know where you want to meet, and we'll come to you.

Jennifer and Mark e-mailed:
Greg,

We haven't met, but I am Holly and Sharley's cousin Jennifer. I grew up with her in Dallas and have seen her strength thru many challenges and heartaches as well as happy laughs, dance-offs, sing-alongs, family trips to lakes, cabins, beach reunions…too many to count. I was so happy to hear that you two found each other and clearly by your note, you will help her move beyond this next challenge. My love and prayers to all of you, and may each day bring improvement for Holly. She is a strong one, and with the love of you, Sharley, Dave, and those above…I have to believe she will get past all of this.

Thank you so very much for including me in this update. Please know your cousins in Atlanta are praying hard!

From: Payan, Gregory
Sent: Friday, April 25, 2014, 9:09 p.m.
Subject: Holly Friday Update

All:

Tired update from Long Island today, but a positive one. Our surgeon came in early today. As mentioned, he doesn't mince words. While last night he refused to categorize the situation as optimistic, I caught him on my way in this morning, and he was positive.

He said he came in early to check on her. Her eyes were closed, and she's still intubated. Nonetheless, he asked for two thumbs up and got it. He asked her to wiggle her toes, and he got it. He said these were complex neurological functions she performed, and that's positive. In his words, "We're in the game."

Truly, that was the best news of the day. He checked on her again later, saw the response he wanted, and left. But for the most part, Holly was uncomfortable with her bed and her breathing tube for much of the day. She got excited and tried to talk with me when she saw me, but I just calmed her down and told her it was all OK. I pretty much stayed out of eyeshot the rest of the day so she could rest.

They bumped up her sedation a bit, and when I left a few moments ago, she was running a slight fever. The rest of the day, her responsiveness was pretty lethargic but not cause for concern, I am told. None of this is abnormal. If I wanted to classify it, she appeared more like someone who wanted to rest (think about trying to wake a tired partner who just wants you to leave), as opposed to being unresponsive. She was resting peacefully when I left. She's been through a lot this week, and not much was done today. Again, the biggest thing to be optimistic about was the opinion of her surgeon, who was pleased this morning. I will take that with me as I try to sleep tonight, and I hope you all do as well.

As far as what you can do, by the end of tomorrow, I'll get a note out with some details. It likely will be cards, a photo (if you have one), and socks. I think it would cheer her up as she starts to become responsive to have a different pair of fun socks each day. Extra points if you write a message on the soles of the feet so the nurse can tell her whom the socks are from, along with maybe something fun or inspirational. Hospital socks/booties are lame, and I think she'd appreciate fun socks. Her room is loaded with machines, so there's not much room for anything else.

I fear that too many of you are praying for a woman prone in a hospital bed. So let's try to spin it the next few days. Holly and I drove up the Black Sea coast of Turkey over New Year's, and I took a bunch of silly pictures on my phone of her dancing in our hotel room before we went out to celebrate the New Year by a bonfire. She is vivacious and radiant and beautiful, so let's try to remember that when she's next in your thoughts and prayers.

Thanks and love to you all.

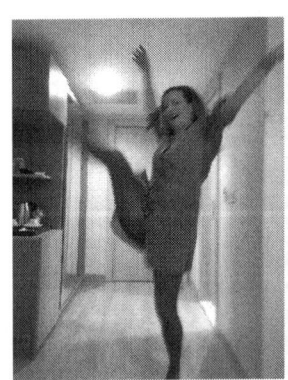

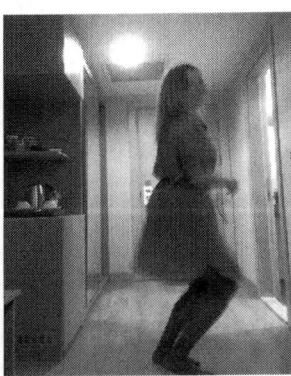

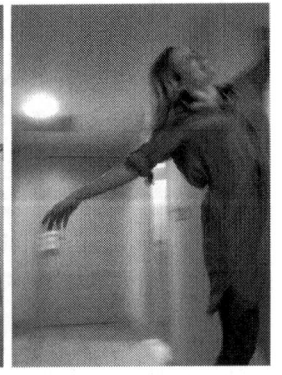

Holly being Holly and expressing her exuberance with a dance before a New Year's party in Turkey.

Please Stay

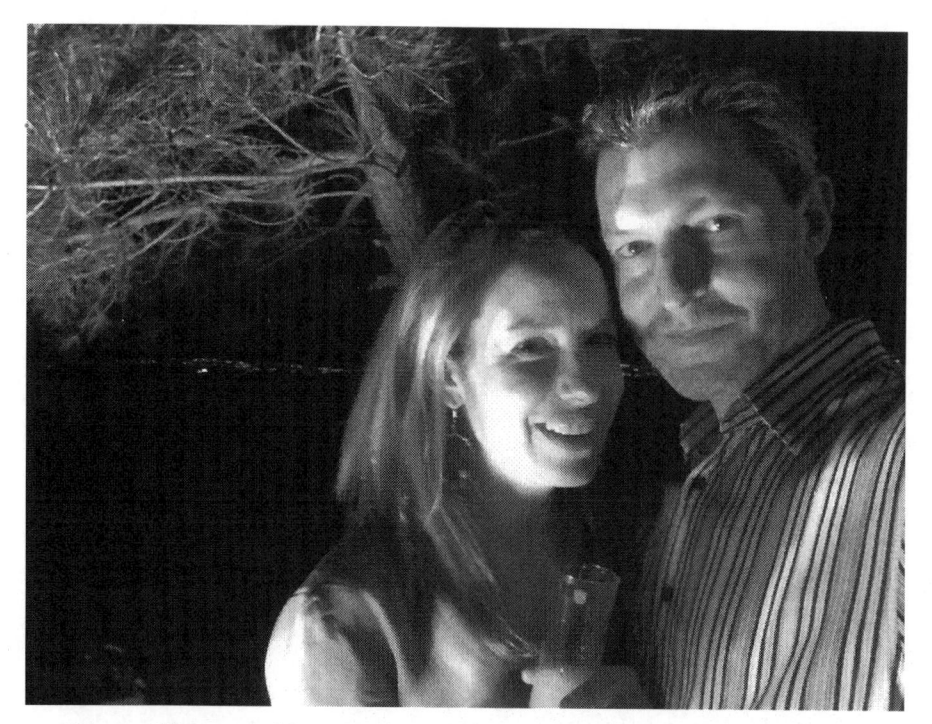

We are illuminated by a New Year's Eve bonfire in Sinop, Turkey, 2013.

Demy e-mailed:
Hi Greg,

Thanks again for the update. What wonderful news! My heart is singing, and these past few days as I have been praying, hoping, and pleading for Holly, I also close my eyes and I think of her wonderful spirit and smile, her beautiful dimples, her heartfelt laugh, her love of life and food and wine. I think of her love of the waves and Bruno Mars! Our quest last summer to go see him and her little boogie dance. Little moments flash, and I smile and laugh and tear up—lots of emotions for my wonderful, strong friend. Thanks for reminding us to not lose sight of all that. I hold that Holly close and dear to my heart…But good to remember!

I'm so relieved and thankful today and will continue to hold hope and pray and keep you all in my thoughts.

Mary e-mailed:
Hey Greg.

It's Holly's cousin Mary in New Orleans. I am and will be saying many, many prayers for all of you, especially tomorrow! Please kiss Holly for me, and we will all be looking forward to good news tomorrow! Holly is strong and will get through this! Until then, whatever you need, we are all here for you! Lots and lots of prayers and love your way!

I LOVE the news and these pics! Such a ballerina! Yaay, Holly! Keep moving your toes and fingers…

Can't wait to see you in person soon. Xoxoxo

Holly has described me in the past as "steady" or "solid." While not the most exciting of compliments, it meant a lot to me. My parents instilled a sense of duty, as well as resolve, in me. Holly and I were not married, but I believed in "richer or poorer," "for better or for worse," and "in sickness and in health." All those words carried deep meaning within me. I had so many hours in the hospital alone with my thoughts and could not help wondering what our lives would be after her aneurysm rupture. I was trying to come to grips with the idea that I may came out of this tragedy as a tortured soul, potentially taking care of her on a daily basis. I knew that, regardless of what happened and what we became, I wasn't going anywhere. I was ready to accept what fate had in store.

DAY 6—HOLLY SPEAKS
April 26, 2014

THE NEXT MORNING, MY PHONE rang at 7:00 a.m. The time of the call and the area code, 516, made me fear the worst. I knew the call was from the hospital. I answered with my heart in my throat.

Despite fearing the worst, I got great news. I was told that Holly's breathing tube had been removed, and she was asking for me. I said I was already dressed and would be there shortly. Holly could speak for the first time since her ride to the second hospital where she was intubated. I had no idea what she would say or what to expect.

7:14 a.m.
Shar texted me:
Morning.

I replied:
Why are you up so early?
Having a coffee here.
Then shower,
then collecting pix for her wall and munchkins for ICU staff.
Should be there around 8:15.
Her breathing tube is out, and she's talking!

Joan e-mailed:
Hi Greg,

I am Aunt Joan to Holly. Her dad and I are cousins, and my family and I watched Holly grow up into a beautiful young woman as they lived in Arlington and we live in Dallas. My husband, Walter, and our children, Jennifer, Andrew, and Mary Lynn, grew up with Holly and Sharley, and we spent many birthdays, Thanksgivings, Christmases, and Fourths of July together. Thank you for the lovely photos. We will get on your request and will write to Sharley as well. Both those girls have grown into fabulous women. I can tell that Holly has made a wonderful choice in you. God bless. Both of you are in our prayers. Thanks so much for the update.

Cynthia e-mailed:
Greg,

Those photos made my night yesterday. Love seeing Holly doing what Holly does best: dancing and being silly.

How's Holly doing today? Praying, praying, praying for continued improvement. My heart feels lighter after the more positive news from yesterday.

Keely e-mailed:
Hi Greg,

Thanks so much for calling, for your updates via e-mail, and for these pics!

I, like everyone, have been obsessively thinking about Holly. I think about her smile, her voice, her laugh, her insight, and HER DANCE MOVES! Like for real, I've been admiring them for years. So these pictures make me so happy.

You are doing so great. I know you might not feel like you are b/c the past six days have been just totally traumatic, but from my perspective and everyone I know, you know, and Holly knows, you are a superhero. THANK YOU, THANK YOU, THANK YOU!

Please Stay

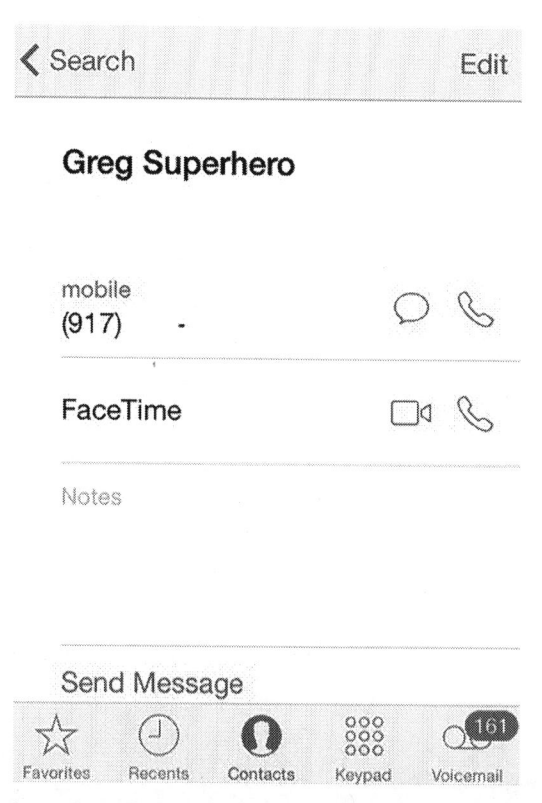

> **Greg Superhero**
>
> mobile
> (917) -
>
> FaceTime
>
> Notes
>
> Send Message
>
> Favorites Recents Contacts Keypad Voicemail (161)

Holly's friend Keely sent this image of my entry on her iPhone contact list. It made me laugh and gave me a bit of extra strength, letting me believe I might be a little stronger than I felt.

Marjorie e-mailed:
Hello Shar and Greg!

Couldn't have been more pleased yesterday to receive such positive news. That Holly is so strong!

A pair of socks is the most fabulous idea, and I can she see her smiling about that. I will be on the hunt!

Shar, we haven't met, but I met Holly years ago in Montauk, and we have often spent time sipping some sunset cocktails, dining out, sharing a house, or doing yoga (she was kind enough to do a yoga lesson for my husband/then boyfriend and me—and boy did he need guidance). The way I describe Holly is pure light.

I just wanted to send some love and support to both of you. I can only imagine how challenging this week has been for you. Holly is lucky to have you both!

I've gone out to Ditch to say prayers for Holly a couple of times. One time the ocean was too choppy to surf and the other too smooth—like a lake. I am guessing the waves are waiting for her to recover to be prime!

I don't know the first thing Holly said when her breathing tube was removed, as it happened just after dawn. If I had to guess, I'd say she asked for me. I arrived around breakfast, and Sharley came shortly after lunch. When I arrived, she simply greeted my arrival with a "Hey, honey. What's up?"

Holly, anxious to make up for lost time when she had a breathing tube down her throat refused to stop talking for much of the day. Most of it made sense, and some of it didn't, but her brain was working, and she was recognizing people, if not totally understanding what she'd gone through and where she was.

11:10 a.m.
Shar texted me:
What's up?

I replied:
All good.
She's still chatting and moving,
though she is a bit scared.

Please Stay

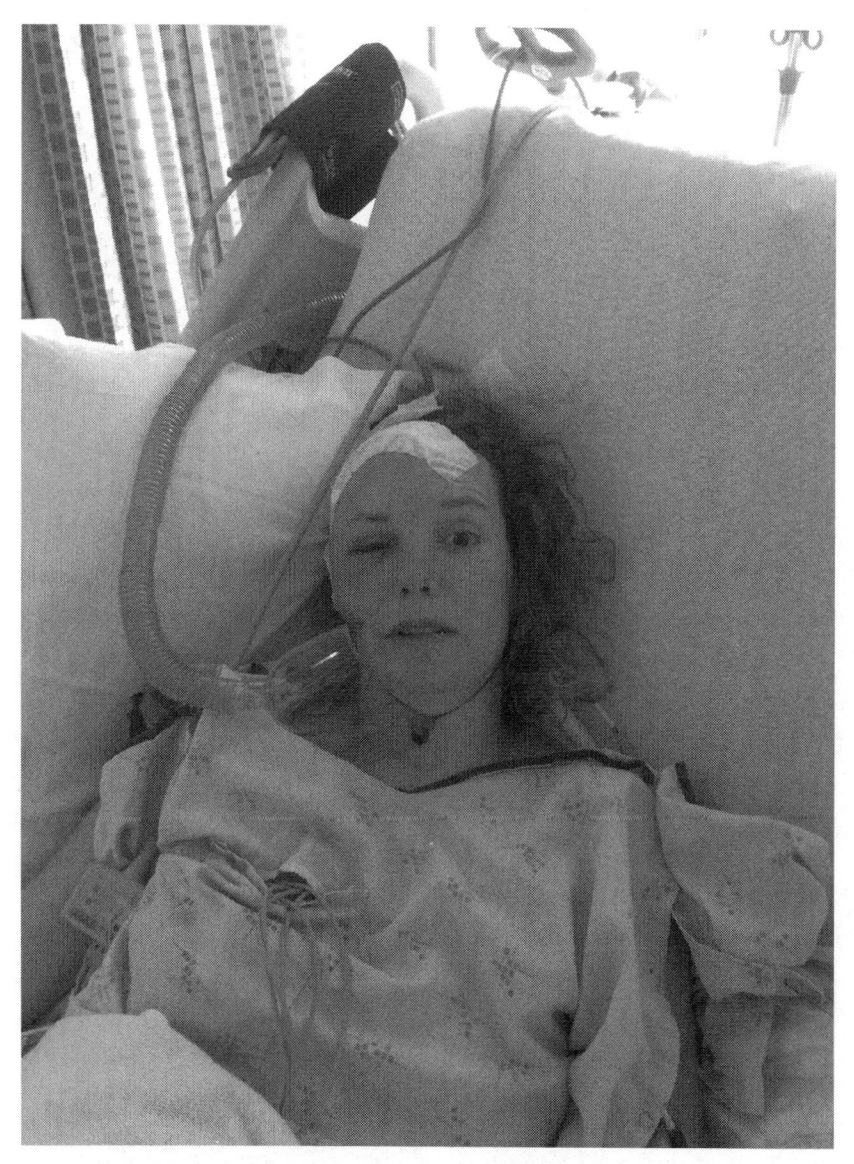

Sharley's photo of Holly after her breathing tube was removed.

2:44 p.m.
Shar texted me:
Hope you're enjoying lunch.
She is finally asleep!
They are sonogramming her legs
to make sure she doesn't have any clots

> **I replied:**
> I just got a bagel.
> Coming back now

Shar texted:
I don't know if there is room in here!
Take a longer break. Go outside!

> **I replied:**
> Already here.
> Nurse said to wait outside the door.
> Will come in when they are done.

Shar texted:
I told them she seems to be a little more disoriented.
They said they were aware.

4:04 p.m.
I texted Shar:
Things seem a bit better.
From eight to eleven, she was good.
Her confusion started around when you arrived,
and it's been up and down.
I think she's a bit better since I came up.
I talked with her nurse for twenty minutes,
and she said do not worry.
Only if motor skills go or she starts to slur.
I really think this is OK,
and I am a worrier.

Shar replied:
:)
What time ya leaving
for your outing with your friends?
R ur parents still here?

I replied:
Folks still here.
I am thinking of leaving around 6:30 or so.

Krista e-mailed:
Dear Greg and Sharley,

Your daily updates are so very welcome and appreciated, Greg. In this one, I felt you exhale a little for the first time. There is certainly a long and challenging road ahead, but there is palpable hope. May you both find ways to take care of yourselves and one another amid these trying days.

From the beginning, I have been imagining Holly—and holding her in the light—at her brightest and most radiant. It is hard to imagine her any other way. She is strong and wise and positive; I have no doubt that such enduring qualities, even in her fragile and sedated state, have been a huge component of the "miracles" so far. She will rise and dance again; my heart knows this to be true.

Please let me know how/where I can send socks. What a fantastic idea.

When people talked about Holly's strength, they weren't discussing a facade. Not even close. Nor was it armor protecting her from what she really felt. It was real, every bit of her strength—along with her lust for life. What made it all the more admirable was that such passion remained after she'd endured what may have broken others who had experienced similar loss and heartbreak. In spite of losing her mother and her husband, she was still fierce.

There is a quote that makes it around the Internet these days in a meme. It says, "Fate whispers to the warrior, 'You cannot withstand the storm.' The warrior whispers back, 'I am the storm.'" I think of Holly whenever I see it.

From: Payan, Gregory
Sent: Saturday, April 26, 2014, 7:41 p.m.
Subject: Holly Saturday Update

All:
Today, good and righteous seemed to win over circumstance. Holly woke up early, and the respiratory therapist wanted to remove her intubation tube. He took it out around 7:00 a.m., and immediately she began to talk and ask for me. Once I arrived, we proceeded to chat for the better part of eleven hours, despite the fact that she desperately needed sleep but could not get comfortable. It was a funny, weird, strange, scary day, but everyone says we should all be encouraged.

    She was able to drink some water and even had some dinner (think baby food) that she probably ate too fast; it made her a bit sick. She is having some vasospasms, which is normal, but they can also be a precursor to a stroke. When an aneurysm ruptures and blood is released into the brain, it winds up where it shouldn't be. This loose blood can land on another vessel, causing it to spasm and possibly close down. This can cause a stroke because the blood supply is cut off.

    She also has what appears to be ICU psychosis, and her heart function is still not optimal after the multiple traumatic situations, but again, it was a good day. As for the ICU psychosis, it's not uncommon, but it's scary. She is hallucinating and paranoid. She's not frightened terribly, but it's really weird behavior. To give you an idea of the day, here are some of the funnier things she said:

- I can't bring in my dissertation for the hospital staff to read. I think they'd have trouble with Mirabai and Hadewijch.
- Tolstoyism isn't really a religion; it's more a social movement.

- Can I touch your face? I only have one eye (the other is swollen), and I have no depth perception.
- I'm really having trouble with one of my religion classes. They just don't get it.
- I think my big old butt knocked out an important tube when I shifted.
- We gotta break outta this place. I'm serious. We need a plan.
- "What kind of socks should I have people send?" I asked. Holly replied, "I need smart socks. I need to be successful in my field."

Some of the stranger things she said, likely brought on by the ICU psychosis:

- Can you get me that beer on the shelf?
- I need you to e-mail the consulate in Thailand. I think we're being spied on.
- I think a woman just came in here and stole your iPad.
- There's a man looking through the window, and he's pointing at me.

Hopefully, you get the picture. She is terribly uncomfortable and just can't rest, which makes me sad. They can't put her on sedatives or any heavy painkillers. She has a headache, and she's sore. She's already sick of her bed and is limited in the positions she can stay in. She seems to like company thus far, but we'll hold off on visitors for some time.

Following up, if you want to send something, cards are good. You can also send one photo (five-by-seven size with a caption on the back) if you have one and one pair of fun socks (just up to the ankle, please) with your name and inspiration or quote on the sole, written in marker. No obligation whatsoever, but if you want, please send away, and I will make sure Holly gets them.

There always remains the threat of complications in the coming hours/days/weeks, but she remembered everyone whose name we brought up (just a few today). Everyone she saw, she remembered. She got plenty of things wrong, but they were not deemed critical. She knew her name, her birthday, Barack Obama, Mitch McConnell, the year, etc. She had a tough time grasping that she was in Long Island and why, but she thought she'd had a migraine headache earlier this week. They want her to know that she had a ruptured aneurysm, so they were blunt, and it scared her a bit. She looked at me kind of sadly and wanted me to answer the doctor's questions or instruct him to give her a different diagnosis. But we told her, and she accepted it well.

Pray for her to be able to rest comfortably through the night. It's what she needs most. We can worry about baby steps forward tomorrow, but she really needs a good night's sleep.

Her personality was Holly. She was smart and funny and beautiful. Think a really happy, sleepy drunk who's a bit paranoid. That was Holly today, the first day out of six harrowing, dangerous days. It was encouraging.

In all, it was a very good day, I am told, and I have to trust the professionals.

Thanks for all the continued love and prayers.

Keely e-mailed:
Greg,

It sounds like a funny, weird, strange, scary day, for sure. I hope Holly and you and Shar can get some good rest tonight. I wish she could have painkillers. I'm going to go shopping right now on Etsy and see if I can't find some good socks. You're amazing, just like Holly! She's even smart with her ICU psychosis.

John e-mailed:
Greg,

I posted parts of your update to my website, and a lot of my readers have had some experience with ICU psychosis. They all suggested that if you know a massage therapist, have them come in and massage her and play soft but complicated music (classical, etc.), and that will help her mental state. In previous threads, one of the most important things they said you could do was simply hold her hand. I've taught nonverbal communication for close to twenty years, and I cannot tell you how much I concur. Human touch is so very important. Won't go into boring discussions about it, but really, holding her hand and human touch are just so, sooo important.

I am also thrilled that you sound so much better mentally.

Stew e-mailed:
So happy for you both. You made Erin, Ella, and I head to mass on Saturday night.

8:37 p.m.
I texted Shar:
I just left.
Michaela is her night nurse.
She and Holly were talking about the beach.
She got some orders for some IV Tylenol from the doctor.
Hopefully this will help Holly to rest.

9:55 p.m.
Shar texted me:
How is your night going?

I replied:
Good. Relaxing.
Will call nurse station at 10:30 or 11.
Love you.

Shar texted:
Friends over?

I replied:
Yep.
Just talking and drinking.
Doing OK.
Trying to get my strength up.
How are you?

Shar texted:
Oh good.
I am home eating dinner
and so happy to be drinking a glass of wine!
I am happy to call her nurse at 10:30 and text you.
Sound good?

I replied:
Sure.
Thanks.
Likely going in around 8:30 tomorrow,
once my folks get back from church.

Shar texted:
No problem.
How about I come pick you up at 8:30?

I replied:
Sounds good

Shar texted:
I have your car,
so your wish is my command, sir.

I replied:
OK.
Let me know she's OK at 10:30.
Make sure you rest after you call.

Shar replied:
OK for all things.

During Holly's crisis, text messages and updates between Sharley and me were often monotonous, mundane, and even boring when looked at in retrospect. Sharley and I functioned as a team when Holly was sick. When someone was at Holly's bedside and the other wasn't, we wanted to know what was happening. We needed to celebrate the good as a team and also share the bad. We leaned on each other daily, even hourly, to make the most awful of situations just a bit more bearable. Every day seemingly began and ended with us checking in with each other, and we spoke many times in-between.

This book has only a sampling of our hundreds of messages to each other. We always checked in with each other to give strength before starting each day anew, and we always checked in with each other at day's end to make sure we knew Holly was OK—and that we were too. These texts were critical, because often one of us was alone at Holly's bedside when she was in pain or while she slept, with only the beeping of machines keeping us company for hours on end. The texting always made me feel loved, among family, and less alone. They were critical during those days in the ICU.

Demy e-mailed:
Hi Greg!

Wow, what a day. Your e-mail made me laugh, smile, tear up, hold my breath, and jump for joy. All emotions at once. Eleven hours. Incredible. The ICU psychosis sounds scary for Holly—and you and Shar. It seems like it's another "normal" part of the process. But overwhelming nonetheless, given the other parts. I am so glad she is in such an expert and caring facility.

It's incredible that almost six days later, she is the Holly we know, and the things she brought up made me smile so hard! I'm hoping and praying for strength as Holly lets the news sink in about her condition—and above all, rest for her tonight. She is in my thoughts at all times.

Thanks as always for your thoughtful e-mails. Card, picture, and socks will arrive from me—I love that you thought of the socks…I am on the hunt for the perfect socks for my dear friend.

Wanda e-mailed:
All good signs.
Sending much love.
She's back.
Yaaay!

11:51 p.m.
I texted Shar:
You check in?
Our girl OK?

Shar replied:
Report from her nurse:
Holly slept for almost an hour once I left.
The Tylenol drip helped.
Most recently,
she is awake again.
She sees people walk by and gets disturbed.
Neuro exam's good
She told Michaela
to tell you and me if we called that she loved us!
Our girl is def OK!
Get some rest.
Michaela said she is all good!

I texted:
Awesome.

Shar replied:
:)
Xoxo

A group of my childhood friends came to my parents' house that evening to watch a basketball game with me. We didn't share anything too emotional. They didn't offer any advice. I didn't vent my fears and frustrations. We simply watched basketball and drank beer while talking a bit clinically about the situation. We had some laughs. Because I've known these friends for decades, little needed to be said. They showed their support by being there when I needed them. That was more than enough. It was a small break and gave me a bit of a lift for the long, grueling days that would follow.

Part 2
Healing and Complications

DAY 7 — STRUGGLING
April 27, 2014

7:01 a.m.
Shar texted me:
Morning.

> **I replied:**
> Morning.
> Checked in at the hospital earlier.
> All vitals good,
> but she was calling out a bit through the night.
> Going to walk there now.
> Need exercise and sun and music.
> It's about an hour walk.
> Will meet you there.
> Xoxoxo

Shar texted:
Are you sure?
Can I call you a cab and pay for it?
Just trying to think of fastest option!

> **I replied:**
> No, she's OK.
> I told them to tell her I would be there soon.

Shar texted:
OK, no prob.
I spoke with Michaela
regarding the noticing everybody walking by the room—
she told me this happens after a major event like this.
Holly is unaware of her surroundings and scared.
They are very good at comforting her.
She also keeps talking of breaking out
And her concept of time is skewed also.
I told her we would be there in morning as soon as we could.
This is good—her spirit and stubbornness are there!

I replied:
OK.
It's beautiful out.
This walk will help me.
Struggling a bit today.

Shar texted:
Enjoy the fresh air.
I will be over nine-ish.
I will bring you a bagel with cream cheese and coffee.

I replied:
K. Love ya.

Shar texted:
We can do hard things together.
Love you...

9:09 a.m.
Shar texted me:
Breakfast order, please?
I'm downstairs.

Please Stay

I replied:
Not hungry.
Here with her.

Shar texted:
How is she?
Glad you made it!

I replied:
Not as good as yesterday.
Real tired.
Respiration up.
They are giving her another CT scan
I will take a walk
and say a prayer by the life rock
when you arrive.

Outside the entrance to the hospital was an enormous, oddly shaped, white rock dubbed the "Life Rock." It was 20 feet from the building entrance, having been donated by someone many years before with a plaque on top of it noting it was there for "positive energy." Throughout Holly's ICU stay, I said a quick prayer by the rock every time I entered or left the building.

Kathryn e-mailed:
Hi Greg,

I don't know you, but I know Holly, and thus I know you must be a wonderful, compassionate person. I heard through the grapevine that you wanted memories, thoughts, and love for Holly to read to her as she fights to stay with us. I hope you will share this with her.

Holly,

Can I call you that? I guess it's been almost ten years now since you were my teacher at Arlington High, so "Mrs. Hillgardner" seems a little antiquated, but Holly sounds unfamiliar too. I know it's been a long time. I think about you a lot though. I work for a nonprofit dedicated to fighting cancer now, and I reflect often on the story you told us in that first yoga class I had with you at Arlington High. I remember your husband, who died of liver cancer when you were so young in Texas, and his fight. What strength and poise you had. You were the first person I had known that truly embodied the phrase "the world is a reflection of you."

I see death all the time in what I do, mostly from cancer, something you know all too well. You can probably see it right now, too. But I don't think it's your time. There is still so much to fight for, so many students, so much love and compassion to spread. The world needs you, and you have the fight to come back. I know you can; I know you will.

Growing up in Arlington wasn't always easy for me, but you made it easier. I always thought of you as a success story, a story beyond the grief and sadness of this world. You are that and so much more to me. I remember in yoga class how you encouraged Kandrea and I in our Cirque du Soleil-style moves and how you taught us what *savasana* really meant and what it was to clear your mind. I loved that class, and I loved you. You have touched so many people—*you aren't done yet.*

Where I work, we do a cross-country bicycle ride to raise money for cancer. The riders are college students with a passion to fight the disease. Each ride, each meeting, they do ride dedications for those fighting cancer or other diseases. We will ride for you this week, Holly. We're fighting for you.

11:40 a.m.
Shar texted me:
I'm back in room.
She has a fever, but they will treat it.
Waiting on respiratory.
She is sleeping but breathing fast,

thirty-eight to forty breaths a minute.
Should be around twenty.
Will keep you updated.
Kicked back out for a few minutes,
They have to draw a bunch of labs, fever of 102.4.

> **I replied:**
> OK.

2:11 p.m.
Shar texted me:
Come see me up the hill at the playground.
I am breathing deep for her in the sunshine b/c she cannot.

> **I replied:**
> OK.
> Meet you there.

Shar texted:
K

Kris e-mailed:
Hello, Greg and Sharley,

I really appreciate the updates. I have to tell you an amusing story. I was talking to my husband about Holly on Friday, and he said, "That's weird. The political blog I follow has updates about a girl with a brain aneurysm too—what are the odds?" Well, after more talking, we realized that it was the same girl! It made us both realize that the world really can be a large community of friends who care for each other. My husband and I move in very different worlds—he is a computer scientist, and I am a sociologist—and this is the first time our two circles of friends have meshed. (We just got married seven months ago.) I just thought I would tell you this story as a way of saying how Holly has such an incredible ability to bring people together and touch people's lives. I am sure that the two of you already know that well, but it's worth repeating.

3:31 p.m.
I texted Shar:
At Italian restaurant.
Ordered clams.
Listening to opera.
Drinking wine.
Terribly sad yet happy to be out for a few.
I promise to be strong for her when you leave tomorrow.
Xoxoxo

Shar replied:
So happy to read this!
Enjoy a lunch to yourself.
Finishing decorating the walls in her room with pix!

From the moment Holly was admitted, I felt it was vitally important to humanize her for her nurses. In no way at the hospital did we feel that she was ever treated with anything but the best of care, but it was important for me to know that her caregivers knew who they were taking care of. She needed to be seen as a complete person and not just a patient hooked up to monitors and tubes and represented by words on a chart or numbers on a machine. I wanted them to see who she was through a collection of photos.

There are strict rules in the ICU about what can be put into a room or how it can be decorated. Flowers, among other things, were not allowed. Pictures were. Holly had lived a wonderful life, traveling any moment she could. I wanted to put as many photos up as I could of a woman with a big smile and bouncy, curly hair traveling throughout the world. When she was crying out in the middle of the night or being visited by nurses, they could see who they were taking care of. She wasn't just another patient; she was Holly. They could see these photos, see a young woman traveling the world, and ask questions. They could engage her at 3:00 a.m. when she had a headache and asked for pain medications and speak to her person to person, as opposed to nurse to patient. When she was sad or could not sleep, her nurses might ask her where the photo was taken of Holly with a monkey on her head, or of her in a rice paddy, or when she posed in front of a barren landscape of white snow somewhere in the world that might not be clear at first glance.

I feel this was one of the best things Sharley and I did. Holly still would have received wonderful care, but I think it made a difference. I am eternally indebted to her caregivers, but it was important to me for her caregivers to see 'Holly', and not just a patient on their daily rounds.. Maybe it did not make any difference. But maybe it did.

There were pictures all over the wall of her ICU room. It made us happy. It made visitors happy, and hopefully it made Holly happy. And as for her nurses and doctors, they knew the person they were caring for and nursing back to health on a slightly deeper level. And that was the ultimate goal.

I e-mailed Cynthia and Demy:

Thanks so much for the offer to come by. I will take you up on it, but I'm just not sure how best to schedule yet. Shar leaves tomorrow, and Holly has not had a good day. She's very lethargic and running a fever. Her respiration rate is higher than it should be, and she had a CT scan, which they did not like regarding the vasospasms and potential serious complications that could arise. They might raise her blood pressure to combat them, which is not good for her heart, which still remains compromised. Lots of moving parts, as you can see, but neuro signs do remain good.

Tomorrow she will be under general anesthesia in the a.m. and undergo an angiogram. That will confirm that the clip is solidly in place and blood flow around the brain is good.

If you can keep your schedules a bit open, I can ring you both tomorrow, and we can see what will work on Tuesday and Wednesday. Thank you so, so much.

Demy replied to me:
Thanks for the update. I'm sorry to hear about CT scan. I'm glad they are constantly monitoring, and I hope the outcome will be positive as day progresses and tomorrow. She's in my thoughts. I hope as the day progresses the fever subsides. Hope and prayers!

I'm on standby! And I will keep my Tuesday open and Wednesday until I have to teach open—so both days as indicated are at your disposal...

I responded:
Thank you. I'm trying to let go, so I can make it through the coming days and weeks. She's receiving the best care. Since they are monitoring everything, they keep us aware of everything, and it can be overwhelming. I am sharing so you are aware too. You guys will be rock stars when you're here with her, and I will be here too. I just need to get away every now and again to maintain my sanity.

<u>**6:11 p.m.**</u>
I texted Shar:
Fever broke.
She's sleeping.
Respiration down.
Some things to like.

                                                     Shar replied:
                                                           Yahoo!

From:	**Payan, Gregory**
Sent:	**Sunday, April 27, 2014, 9:19 p.m.**
Subject:	**Holly Sunday Update**

All:

Today was a hard day. After waking up early, I figured I might as well walk to the hospital. It's only three miles, and along with being sleep-deprived, I'm exercise deprived. Popped on the headphones, took off, and picked up some munchkins for the hospital staff and a *New York Times*, some of which I hoped to read to Holly.

After a good cry (listening to Eva Cassidy on my walk in), I got to see her. Her breathing was labored, and she was really sleepy. It was a pretty big change from yesterday. I had checked in when I woke this morn, and she was still restless and hallucinating, so I was kind of expecting a day similar to yesterday, which was not the case. Today was nothing like yesterday.

I think "smooth recovery from brain injury" is not something this world will ever know. With no reference point, you expect a trajectory to remain the same, and when it's not, it's a punch in the gut, but sadly...sort of normal, according to the professionals. It's just that you go crazy. I sit with her and hold her hand and watch as she sleeps and breathes. You see her cough and silently hope she can get the phlegm into her mouth, so she can spit it out, or hope she swallows it, but you don't want to see her choke, and you watch this for way longer than you should, over and over, and then you hear the doctors and nurses talking and saying her respiration rate is forty and should be twenty, and they call for a respiratory therapist, but the therapist is intubating someone, so you wait and suffer for her and wonder when he will arrive and how long intubations take—you want him there, checking on Holly. Then another doctor comes in and yells her name when she just wants to rest, and you want to say, "Shhhhh! She needs her rest," and then he's giving her commands to raise her arms, and she does it really slowly, and you wonder, oh no, is that a sign that she's regressing, or is it just because she had traumatic brain surgery a few days ago and all the poor girl wants to do is sleep? And why are they yelling? And then she raises her arms, and the doctor turns and says, "She looks good." And you realize that it's only been a few hours, and you have all day to watch scenes like this play out over and over, and…you…slowly…lose…your…mind…

Holly did take a small step backward today, but she's peaceful right now. Another CT scan looked good. (These are big, so that's comforting.) She had a fever most of the day (102.4), but it broke around five o'clock. Her respiration was too high for most of the day. It went down but had crept up again when Shar and I left. Her heart is still a bit weak from the incident, but that, too, is not unusual. It lasts five to ten days usually, but it affects how she is treated for other ailments.

She still recognizes everyone and remembers who came to visit her yesterday. She is just soooo lethargic and tired. If this were yesterday, I'd exhale and say, "Whew…this is great." But because it's a step backward, I'm totally upside down. This is the process. I have to get better for Holly, and I will. Please know she's holding her own, according to hospital staff.

Sharley decorated Holly's room today, but she's barely been awake and has not noticed. Pictures of family and friends adorn the walls, and we can't wait for her to be a bit more lucid so we can begin to talk about people and happy memories. We don't have much real estate, but we have some cute photos up.

Also, a few people asked about the Mitch McConnell recognition yesterday. I probably should tell the whole anecdote, because it was kinda cute and probably a fun thing to leave everyone with. I was reading an old copy of the *New Yorker*, and a cartoon of Barack Obama feeding medicine to Mitch McConnell adorns the cover. I was trying to see what Holly could remember, and I said, "You remember Barack Obama, right?" and showed her the cover.

She said, "Of course."

"Who is he spooning medicine to? Mitch…" I said, trying to prod her memory.

And then she stopped me. "Honey."

"Yes?"

"I might have to break up with you," she said.

"Why?"

"I don't know if I can be with someone who doesn't know who Mitch McConnell is."

That brought a smile to my face, and I hope it does for everyone else too. She also made me laugh at one point today when the nurse came in and asked, "Holly, how are you doing?" and Holly replied nonchalantly, "What's uuuuppp?" not unlike the actors in the Budweiser frog commercials back in the day.

That said, Holly is a little sick and a lot tired and lethargic, and her breathing is a bit too heavy. I think we must all just embrace this as part of a long process.

Thanks and love.

Kerri e-mailed:

God bless you, Greg, I'm praying for you, too. It's so hard to watch someone you love suffer.

Kelsi e-mailed:

Greg,

Thank you so much for the continued updates. I know it can't be easy after a long day to sit down and relay it all to us, but we are so, so grateful. And your writing is stunning. I guess I shouldn't be surprised that Holly is in love with a writer. I'm so sorry you have to go through this, and I hope you know that you are in everyone's thoughts and prayers and intentions as well.

My colleague Nat e-mailed:
Greg,

I am so, so, so happy to hear that Holly is on the road to recovery, although these agonizing moments in the process...well, I can't even imagine... Please continue to take care of yourself, as that will be better for you and for Holly. Your notes are amazing, and you and Holly are so lucky to have each other. You must be so overwhelmed, so please know I am here for you for any task you might need help with. All is well at work. Everything is being taken care of, and we are all thinking of you always.

I replied to Nat:
Thanks. I may try to pop into the office this week for a few hours.

I may also ask if you can help and make a fake wedding invitation that I can hang on her wall. She gets nervous when I'm not around and likes to talk about her fiancé. I think once she can be a bit more aware of her surroundings and stable, it would make her happy. Let me see how the next day or two goes. Thanks for holding things together.

Nat responded:
I would love to do a wedding invite for you! Just let me know what you want on it, and I will bust something beautiful out.

Take care, Greg, and don't rush back to work unless you need the break. All is well.

Talk soon.

Francine e-mailed:
Greg,

So thankful for your presence and love of Holly—also the fact she was with you, not in West Virginia, when this happened. Know it must be draining for you and so appreciate your heartfelt updates. Hope you are taking care of you—for you and to be strong for Holly.

You know that no one is ever good enough for someone dear to you. You've exceeded my hope that Holly would find an endearing, but equal, soul mate.

Thinking of you both constantly.

―⁂―

I just knew I could not lose Holly. All my energy, all my love, was directed toward this one person in my world who was my partner, as we had neither children nor plans for any. She was everything to me—part of every day and every plan I made. Nearly everything we did or planned revolved around what we could experience together. To have our life drastically altered, lives we were happily living before her aneurysm, would involve emotional pain I could not even imagine. Even if I would not be a true "caregiver," there had to be fallout after a grade IV brain hemorrhage. Maybe I could adapt and still get joy each and every day, as I had in the past. But Holly…I had huge doubts. Holly is not someone who deals well with restrictions. Some would deem her stubbornness legendary.

The first hurdle would be her job. Her brain had to heal, so she could resume her career as a college professor. It had to heal, and it had to heal soon. The medical professionals implied that a hallelujah chorus should greet every day for the simple fact that she was still breathing after being minutes away from death. It seemed they felt a recovery that might involve only "minimal" deficits was something to be celebrated, but I needed more. For the health of our relationship and her happiness, I needed it all back. Some may say I was being greedy, but I was just being realistic. If she could not teach as a college professor, she could not be happy. If she lost any small bit of her brain function, she would never be OK. If that happened, her happiness would not be possible. And if she was not happy, how could I be?

―⁂―

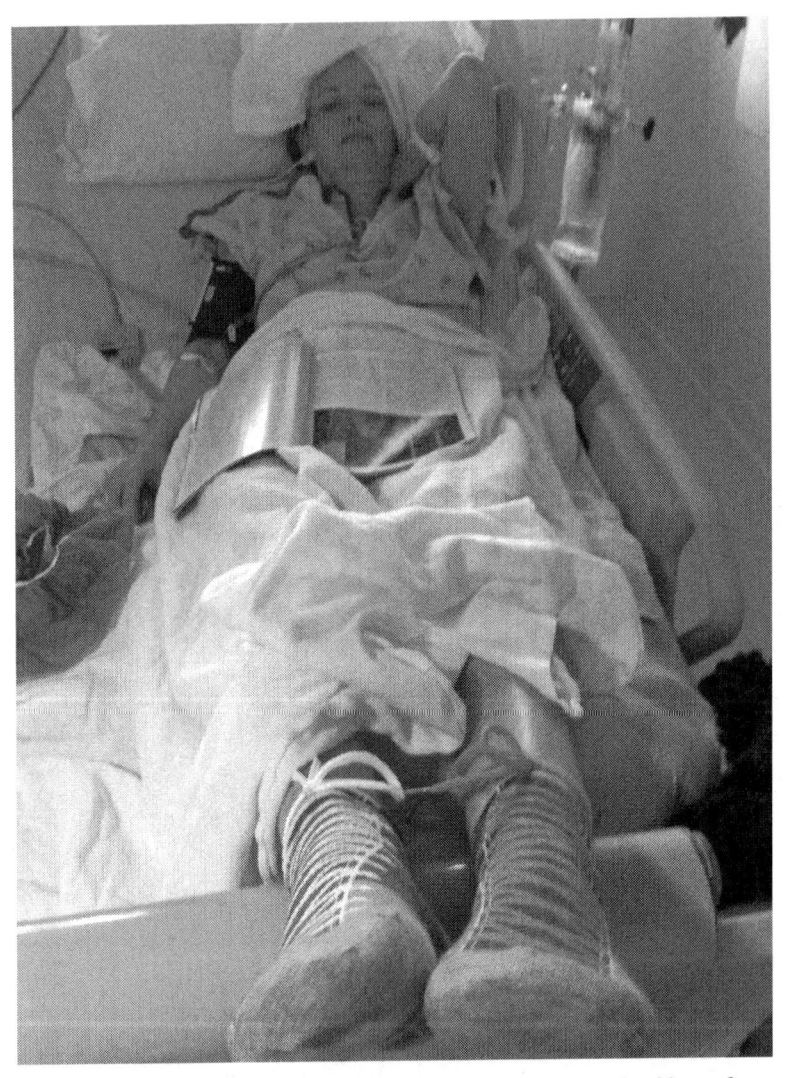

Holly has ice on her head in this photo, the first I took of her after surgery. She's wearing the first pair of socks she received and trying to read a magazine, although she wasn't really up to it.

Karen e-mailed:
Greg,

I just wanted to say how deeply grateful we all are for you. And also how eloquent and bravely honest and vulnerable these notes have been. I expect nothing less from the love of our dear Holly's life. But know that I am blown away and so impressed by you.

Christy and I are going to get some socks and things together tomorrow. We can mail them in or just drop them off at the hospital (with no expectation of getting to see Holly; we want her as calm and rested as possible). Is there anything we can bring or, if sending is better, send for you?

Aileen e-mailed:
Dear Greg,

I'm so sorry today was such a rough day. The road ahead will be filled with a lot of ups and downs. Holly is a strong, amazing woman, and she will make it through this. So will you. Please continue to take care of yourself and nurture yourself in little ways so you can stay strong for the long haul. Maybe a few yoga poses or meditation in the mornings?

You both continue to be in my thoughts and prayers. I anxiously await tomorrow's update for positive news.

10:28 p.m.
Shar texted me:
Dave thinks we might be sharing too many personal details.
this list has a lot of contacts.
When H comes out of all this,
I think she would have maybe wanted more privacy
regarding exact speech, deliriums, etc.
Does that make sense?
Just our humble opinion…
Xoxo

I replied:
OK.
I will dial it back.
It's just been like group therapy.
I am sorry.

Shar texted:
No reason to be sorry at all.
I know it has helped you tremendously. :)
Love you!

April 28, 2014, 12:12 a.m.
I texted Shar:
Still up?
I have the nightly report!
Sleeping on and off, no fever at all.
Her blood gas value was sixty-six,
should be ninety or higher.
They put a non-rebreather O_2 mask on
to bump up her O_2 level.
She is tolerating it fine.
No other issues.
Good night and xo.
Her nurse said she will call you if you need to know anything!

Shar replied:
K, thanks.
G'night.

3:40 a.m.
Shar texted me:
Just woke up and phone was dead.
I was panicking.
Just talked to ICU.

All is well.
No changes from last report.
Xo

I replied:
Xoxox

4:27 a.m.
Shar texted:
:)

Saying "I love you" took on a different meaning when Holly got sick. Prior to her aneurysm, I reserved that phrase mostly for my parents and Holly. But after her aneurysm ruptured, it meant something entirely different. Most often this was noticeable in my interactions with Sharley, but it happened with others as well. Whether via text or on the phone, the support Sharley provided to me was beyond words. Every day of Holly's ICU stay ended with my saying "I love you" to Sharley. It also wound up in my calls or texts with others who loved and supported Holly and me those days. It continues now, years after. Friends who may have never heard me say it before now frequently hear an "I love you" at the end of a call or time spent together or see an "XOXO" at the end of a text exchange.

I love deeper after all this happened and try to say it as often as possible. It flows very naturally to those who sustained me and to others who mean so much to me. It is important for me to say it whenever I can.

DAY 8 — SHARLEY GOES HOME
April 28, 2014

7:37 a.m.
I texted Shar:
Heading over.
Will update you in a bit.

Shar replied:
OK!
Doing some yoga.
I called ICU at 3:30 and texted you—
not sure if you remember.

I texted:
I do.
I crashed around 11:00.
Woke at 2:00 and was up when you texted.
Have a good practice.

Emily e-mailed:
Oh Greg,

I'm sorry you are feeling so down. I know it must seem like you are carrying the world on your shoulders. Please don't forget to breathe. Nobody deserves to get better and to be better than Holly. Please try to decompress and take your mind off of things for one minute so that you can keep going tomorrow.

Thinking of you. And pulling for Holly.

Mindy e-mailed:
Holly,

I don't know how to begin. You gave me my first *C* ever. I was so angry. You made me realize that you gave me a *C* because you expected more out of me. You made me care about my grades beyond just passing a test. You are the reason I joined Lit Mag. You are the reason stayed in Lit Mag. You are the reason I took Advanced Grammar in college. You are the reason I care about English and grammar now. You are the reason that I can diagram sentences in both English and French. I love you, and I am knitting you some socks that will probably be terrible, but they will be specially made for you. I love you.

8:48 a.m.
I texted Shar:
Here.
She is still really sleepy and lethargic,
but vitals are good,
and I saw Dr. Chalif.
He said he likes what he sees regarding the scans.

Shar replied:
YES!
How is breathing?
R they planning angiogram soon?

I texted:
Angiogram planned for this afternoon
Breathing better.
Around thirty breaths a minute.
BP: 130/90

Shar replied:
Do you know what time for the angio?

I texted:
Not sure.

Shar replied:
That is better breathing.
I think I will take a later train today—
would like to be there for angiogram.

I texted:
Let's see when you come in.
She also knew she was in North Shore hospital
and not Thailand.

Shar replied:
Thailand?
When did she think that!

I texted:
Saturday.

Shar replied:
Oh. OK.
I am very happy with Chalif's report!
I am packing up and will be over in a bit.

I texted:
My parents are coming at five to stay
for a few hours
and also to bring brownies for the night staff in ICU.
All peaceful here.
Need a short break when you arrive though.

Shar replied:
Of course.

I texted:
Just got kicked out of her room for a few for more tests.

Shar replied:
Meet you in waiting room.
Be there in two minutes!

Tanya e-mailed:
Dear Greg,

    I am in amazement that you can write these articulate, funny, poignant updates when you, too, must be exhausted and overwhelmed. But I, and all of us at Drew, are grateful. We continue to hold all of you in our thoughts and prayers. Holly may not be able to engage in these wonderful photos you've surrounded her with yet, but she knows she's surrounded with loving faces, and that's important.

    Peace and blessings.

2:10 p.m.
I texted Shar:
Found a pond near hospital on my walk.
Trying to breathe and relax.

Shar replied:
Great idea!
Do some stretching also with breathing!

3:03 p.m.
I texted Shar:
Will be up in ten.
You want a coffee?

Shar replied:
Hazelnut coffee, please—small!
Angiogram will take one to two hrs.
No word on when they are doing it.
I am trying to decide if I should change
my train again
and stay another day.

I texted:
You should go.
I will be all right and will
call you with results once you are on train.

Shar replied:
Not sure if I will be OK
If I'm not here and results are bad

Meghan e-mailed:
Dear Greg and Sharley,

I have been holding my breath, crying, and praying 24-7 that Holly will be OK. To say she is special is an understatement. I don't think I could bear a world without her in it. Please know and tell her how much I love her.

Behind Holly's sweet disposition is one of the strongest and most resilient women I have ever known. Holly is a fighter. I also believe her disciplined Ashtanga practice has given her body and mind an advantage that medicine won't be able to understand. I am feeling optimistic that she is going to kick this aneurysm's butt...and I am picturing a future with her full of laughing till our stomachs hurt; dance parties; chasing Chris Martin around on our surfboards; surfing adventures; and long talks full of depth, intellect, and understanding.

I think Holly has every spiritual or religious sect from around the world praying for her and sending her healing energies. Pam put Holly on the integral prayer list. Johnny (Anthony's friend, John, the fisherman who fell overboard and lived) is sending her his survival vibes. I even have the nuns at the Catholic hospital where I work praying for her.

4:04 p.m.
I texted Shar:
All quiet here.
Still waiting on angio,
which they still say is on the agenda.

Shar replied:
Headed to playground
for sunshine and Vitamin D therapy.

I texted:
K

                            Shar replied:
                            On the way back now.
                            Need anything from cafe?

I texted:
Angio pushed to tomorrow :(
So she can eat now.
They are bringing her food.

                            Shar replied:
                            Knew it.
                            It's b/c I stayed!
                            OK. I will head out then.
                            I think I can still make it to the train station
                            if you take me right now.

Shar had to return home to her husband, Dave, and son, Elliot. I was sick about Holly's situation already, and now I knew I would be worse.

I don't know how people endure situations like this if they are predominantly alone in caring for a loved one. Sharley truly was everything to me in the first week after Holly fell ill, and while I understood that she had to return to Massachusetts, I was heartbroken.

Before she left, we stopped at a small Mexican restaurant near the train station and had one drink, toasting Holly and ourselves for making it through the hardest of weeks.

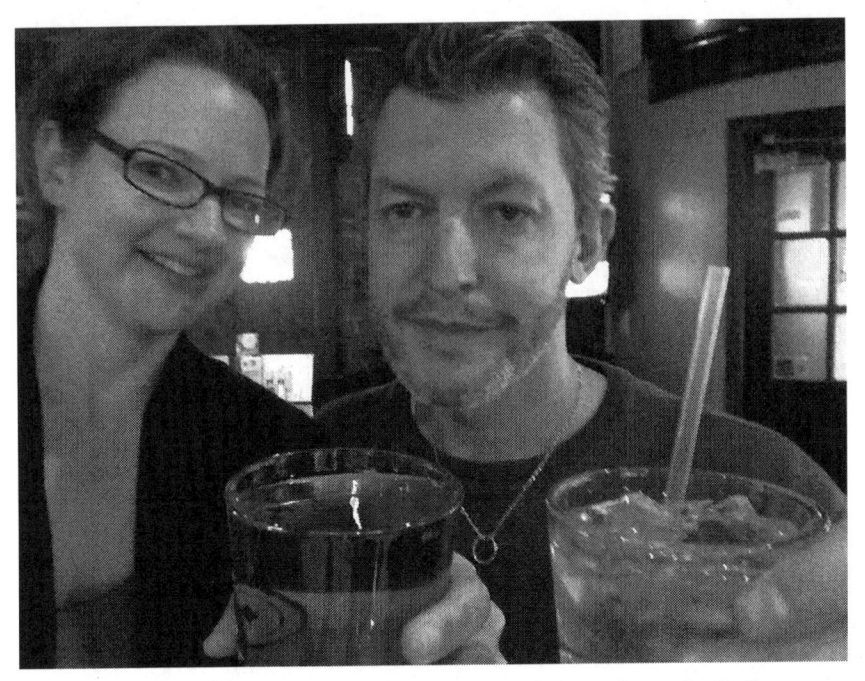

With Sharley, celebrating Holly and making it through the first week. I am wearing Holly's rocksy-proxy ring around my neck.

7:15 p.m.
Shar texted:
On train.
Xoxo.
Quote for you tonight: Peace comes from within.
She is going to be OK!

Mary e-mailed Sharley:
Sharley,

Today we went to Moore Cemetery and visited your mom's grave and said a prayer for Holly…it's such a beautiful gravestone, and Aunt Joan, Uncle Walter, Doug, and I spent some time there on a lovely, sunny, and warm afternoon. The flowers we chose were all white.

Love to you both…Aunt Mary Alice

⁂

From: Payan, Gregory
Sent: Monday, April 28, 2014, 8:28 p.m.
Subject: Holly Monday Update

All:
Today started much like yesterday. Holly was overcome by sleep and lethargy; there was not much happening for most of today. Lots of hand-holding and foot-holding and repositioning of Holly so she could sleep comfortably. No fever, which was great, and her breathing was solid and not labored. We knew they wanted to do an angiogram, but there was an emergency situation in the hospital that they hoped would clear. It didn't, and finally at 4:30, they said they would do the procedure tomorrow. That meant they could feed her.

Holly needed rest after her busy Saturday, but Sharley and I really thought her lethargy was partially due to the fact that she had not eaten in forty-eight hours. We woke her up and told her we could get her some food, and she immediately perked up.

Just a little juice and yogurt, but Holly was ecstatic. She took a sip of orange juice, and then a nurse asked her what her name is.

"Holly," she said.

The nurses explained that they were just making sure she swallowed OK by asking her name in between sips.

Holly then took another sip, and said, "Lynn."

Another sip. "Hillgardner."

Always wanting to do well on tests, I guess.

She noticed all the photos on the wall and was excited and began naming a few people for the nurses and doctors making their rounds. Then a doctor pointed at me and asked Holly who I am.

She said, "Greg Payan. He's the love of my life."

They asked about Shar, and Holly said, "That's Sharley Hillgardner. She's my sister." Then a nurse had the audacity to ask, "Holly, what do you like to do for fun?"

She looked at the nurse as if that were a bad first-date question and said, "Nothing."

The nurse frowned.

Holly said, "Just kidding. I like to travel, and I like to collect degrees."

It was quite an amusing exchange. She said she liked the juice and yogurt much better than the previous afternoon's chicken soup. Being that she had slept for two days and not two hours, she was referencing Saturday's lunch. She chatted a bit more about the photos and traveling and her favorite Dr Pepper shirt that says "Trust me, I'm a Dr.," which I'd brought to the hospital. When told it was Monday, she mentioned that she had to get back to school for her classes, but we keep reorienting her. This is all normal. She remembered where she was born and when she moved to New York and talked a lot about moving to Bethany, West Virginia, where she currently teaches, and fondly described the town.

Holly had her yogurt and her juice and then went to sleep again and was pretty unresponsive for the rest of the day. In all, that ten-minute wake-up and chat—and its confirmation that she's thinking and joking—was a great way to end the day. The fact that Sharley and I saw her surgeon on the way out and he said, "She's doing really good," cemented it. Sharley is convinced that he used the word "miracle."

I do remember him saying this: "If you would have told me we clipped a bayszler (not sure of spelling, as I'm still afraid to look it up) aneurysm and had the complications we did, and she would be in the shape she is today, I'd be jumping for joy."

Since we have discussed that he's not prone to hyperbole, it was a real nice way to end the day.

There is always a lot happening. Tomorrow is a *huge* day, and Sharley and I are scared to death. The angio tomorrow will show that the clip is on perfectly and the blood flow around the brain is what it should be. If it doesn't...I don't want to know what the next step is.

To do the angio, they need to use the only good artery to her brain, since the other tore in the failed coil procedure. If there's a problem...again, I don't want to know. In addition, vasospasms are a constant fear, along with her still-weak heart.

Sharley left tonight to go home to her husband and young child for a few days. Her strength and support have kept me sane, and I am not looking forward to tomorrow without her.

I will keep tonight short. I'm pretty weary. Again, the power of community seems to be working so far, and I will never truly be able to express my gratitude, but thanks again from the bottom of my heart.

Shar replied to my group e-mail:
Neurosurgeon said, "It is a miracle she is OK after all this!" He does not talk to talk; he's a friggin' genius, and he finally looked me in the eye with a smile. I smiled back!

Thank you all for the love and support and prayers. It means so much.
G, you got this angio tomorrow—we are all behind you and her!
Xoxo

Kathryn e-mailed:
Hi Greg,

Thank you again for the continued updates. It means so much to see these each day. I can hardly express what happiness we are feeling here in Texas that Holly continues to progress.

We had one of our team meetings at work, the first since Holly had her aneurysm. I know I only explained this briefly, but I work for a nonprofit organization that raises money for cancer. We do an annual charity bicycle ride from Texas to Alaska each year with a new group of University of Texas–Austin students and cancer fighters. Hopefully that gives you a little perspective on my next comment, which is that I "rode" for Holly last night at the meeting. We do ride dedications at every ride, meeting, etc. for people we know who are fighting cancer or otherwise facing hardship. We will keep riding for her through her healing process.

Ann Marie e-mailed:
Greg,
   Just letting you know I sent this to Holly's sister:

Sharley,
   Let me introduce myself. My name is Ann Marie. I'm Greg's friend Tommy's wife (I believe you met him up at hospital). I have known Greg for the past twenty-six years and love him to death, but Holly makes him that much better! I wanted to thank you for being there to help him deal with all of this. It must be so difficult. I know Holly will be OK. She is strong and healthy and has a lot to live for. I am guessing strength is in the genes somewhere! I knew Holly was special from the first day I met her. She is an interesting, fun, beautiful woman. I have no doubts that she will be back drinking wine in my living room and chatting away with my girls! We will all continue to keep Holly in our prayers.
   Thanks again for being Greg's strength and helping him through this. It means the world to me!

Hope e-mailed:
Hi Greg,
   Just wanted to say that reading your daily Holly updates, they are very heartfelt, and the outpouring of unconditional love you have for her is inspiring and touching. Though I just recently met Holly, I can tell she has a great

personality, quirky sense of humor and is a force of nature (in a good way). My prayers are with Holly, you, and Sharley—and yes, I *did* drop an e-mail note to Sharley. My friend Barbara (a devout Catholic), her prayers are with you and Holly. She will have a mass read for you and Holly at her parish, Church of Our Savior (on Park Avenue in Manhattan). You and Sharley remain strong for each other and for Holly.

9:59 p.m.
I texted Shar:
Just got home.
Sleep pants on, and wine has been poured.
Get home safe.
Will text you at 10:30 after I call nurse.

> **Shar replied:**
> OK.
> Still on train.

10:14 p.m.
I texted Shar:
Holly slept rest of time tonight after you left.
Just spent time holding her hand
and repositioning her.
And delivering brownies to staff.

> **Shar replied:**
> Great!
> Already in Stamford on my ride home!
> Who is night nurse?

I texted:
Melissa—
glasses and long reddish-blond hair.

> **Shar replied:**
> Hmm.
> Have we had her b4?

I texted:
Likely.
She looked very familiar
but not sure if I just saw her on the floor.

Shar replied:
It does sound familiar,
but it is all running together for me.

I texted:
I am so glad you get a few days with your family.
We are fried.

Shar replied:
:)

I texted:
Just called ICU.
They told me to call back in twenty.

Shar replied:
Is Melissa busy,
or there is a problem?

I texted:
Just doing rounds.
Was told she was in with docs.
Not sure if that was with Holly (doubtful)
or with her neighbor,
who my parents said
was brought in in dire straits tonight.

Shar replied:
Oh. OK.
Let me know what you find out!

I texted:
Sit tight for a few.
Will call in ten.

Please Stay

Shar replied:
No problem.

11:36 p.m.
I texted Shar:
Just got off with nurses' station.
Want a text or call?

Shar replied:
Text if it's short.
She OK?

I texted:
Basically, Holly much more alert and doing great.
Nurse was asking me questions about our life
so she can confirm if Holly is speaking
about things correctly and not making things up.
Hol's asking for me a lot.
Melissa wanted to know if we met in France
because Holly keeps talking about that.

Shar replied:
Oh that's great!
Get your rest.
It will be a long day tomorrow.
:)

I texted:
Told her we met in Mexico,
but on Saturday we talked
about going with my parents to France.

Shar replied:
Ahh

I texted:
She's a bit mixed up but much more alert.

> **Shar replied:**
> It's OK.
> Good report!

I texted:
Holly's vitals and awareness really good, they say.

> **Shar replied:**
> You OK?

I texted:
I am good.
Will text you when I arrive in a.m.
Love to you, Dave, and Elliot.
Xoxoox

> **Shar replied:**
> K. Gn, G.

Nancy e-mailed:
Greg,

Still praying, still sending love, still thinking of Hol and you and Sharley constantly. Will send extra prayers for a safe and successful angio tomorrow. And if you need anyone, I know Cynthia and Dee Dee would run to be by your or Holly's side if it would be helpful. I can hear the weariness in your messages, so don't forget about you. Sleep and eat and lean on anyone who is nearby and can help. You need it. Our sweet Holly is going through a wicked recovery (which she is doing amazingly thus far), but you have been through a major trauma, and you need to make sure you are OK too. Holly needs you to be, so promise not to forget about you!

KT e-mailed:
Greg,

After I inquired about a recent Facebook post I had read regarding Holly, Liz was kind enough to forward me your e-mail updates on her.

I want you to know my family and I are praying for her, Sharley, and yourself.

Your e-mails are informative, inspirational, and are helping people more than you realize.

We all go through trials, and reading about Holly's strength and perseverance as she pulls through this gives optimism to those who read your e-mails.

Believe that.

God needs and uses angels to bless others, and your angel is teaching us strength, courage, and determination with every step she takes toward recovery. She will have a story to tell to not only her loved ones and students, but to those she'll one day come in contact with who she doesn't even know at this time, and they'll be blessed all the more after hearing it.

I realize I'm on the opposite coast, but if you need *anything*, please don't hesitate to ask. You're more than a coworker, Greg; you're a friend.

Stay strong, my brother. Godspeed to your beautiful angel.

DAY 9—VASOSPASMS
April 29, 2014

Jess e-mailed:
Dear Holly,

    I just wanted to let you know that you are in my heart and mind.

    One of the things I have always admired (and hoped to emulate) about you is your passion for creating meaning and joy in your life. I know that that zest for life and love of and from so many people you cross paths with will serve you well now. You are a fighter when it comes to life, I know this is true. Don't stop fighting now.

8:33 a.m.
I texted Shar:
Hol resting and good.
She made fun of me when I came in.
Said to the nurse....That's my boyfriend.
He's all right, but I'll keep him.
She's sleeping now.

                                                  Shar replied:
                                                    Oh, that's great.
                                                    Thanks, Greg.
                                               How you doing today?

I texted:
Just praying for a smooth day with the angio.

Shar replied:
Oh yes, of course.
I've already prayed this morning
for him for the procedure,
and my friends know Dr. Chalif's name
and have circulated it out to their friends,
and they're praying too
It will be OK.

I texted:
Xoxo

Shar replied:
Xo

I texted:
Also, no oxygen-assisted mask today.

Shar replied:
WOW!
That's awesome.
Is ur mom with you yet?

I texted:
Mom came.
Could not keep her away.

Shar replied:
Yes!
Oh, ur mom is wonderful—
we are so lucky!
Tell her the goodie bag she made for my trip home
on the train rocked last night!

I texted:
Holly has thrush
but otherwise did great on her checkup.

Shar replied:
Hmm, OK.
Is it bothering her?

I texted:
Bothering her a bit.
Given meds she will swish around in her mouth.
She brushed her teeth this a.m. too.
More progress....

                                        Shar replied:
                                                    Cool!

I texted:
Xoxo

                                        Shar replied:
                   Is 11:00 maybe the time for procedure?

I texted:
They think it will be soon.
But no confirmation on time it will happen.

                                        Shar replied:
                             OK. Who is with you?

I texted:
My mom and Demy.
Won't hear anything for a bit.
Told them to get lunch and go to Life Rock.

                                        Shar replied:
                   OK. Good plan. It's going to be OK.
                      They will be done in an hourish,
and it will be confirming the clip is rock solid,
                                    which we know.
                                      is she scared?

I texted:
She was a bit confused.
Thought that we could go back to
apartment after the procedure.
She had a bad headache and was hungry/thirsty, etc.

They gave her morphine,
so she was in less pain but not as lucid.
She wasn't scared though.
She did great with the occupational therapist.

Shar replied:
Awesome!

I texted:
Please let this next two hours go quickly with good results.
I think it will be a huge step for Holly and you and me.

Michelle e-mailed:
Greg,

I am just receiving all of these e-mails. And again, crying as I read them. I had no idea you were writing them. The power of prayer is amazing. We are all praying today for the procedure to go smoothly, which I am sure it will. I would love to come see you and Holly now that we are back, so please let me know when the best time is.

I love you and am thinking of you guys constantly!

Wondering if you are able to play her music? Music is helpful in healing, especially brain injuries. I can send you some links of music with specific frequencies for healing. Or just play some of her favorites.

Liza e-mailed:
Hi Greg,

When you are ready for the scientific stuff, I found a pretty good site. Basilar just refers to the location (only 5 percent incidence there).

http://www.bafound.org/

Try to rest yourself and stay calm. It sounds like an amazing recovery has begun.

1:11 p.m.
I texted Shar:
Sorry, could not pick up phone earlier.

Shar replied:
Just out of work and was calling to check in.
How is she?

I texted:
Angio good.
Everyone pleased.

Brian e-mailed:
Hope today went well, and I was thinking of both you and Holly. Good luck and keep the faith, brother.

I replied to Brian:
Thanks. Mostly good day. Clean angio, which was the biggest hurdle. Clip on tight, and blood flow good. She is having vasospasms, which is dangerous but not unexpected. Feel pretty OK with today, in the end.

Brian responded:
Awesome! That's great f'ing news, buddy. Stay positive and let me know if you need anything or another night for beers, etc.

From: Payan, Gregory
Sent: Thursday, April 29, 2014, 10:54 p.m.
Subject: Holly Thursday Update

Hey everyone:
Mostly a good day today. There's never a truly good day in this process, but today offered more hope in the journey. Holly got a clean angiogram for the most important things

Please Stay

being monitored. The aneurysm clip is tight, and the blood flow around her brain is good. This was confirmed by the dye injected for the procedure. This was fabulous news. As with every step in this process, the enthusiasm is a bit muted, as the angiogram did also confirm vasospasms in the area of the bleed. This is *not* unexpected, but it's also not good. It means she is at heightened risk for a stroke. That said, they are fully aware and are treating her to prevent that. This process is brutal, but today should be a cause for a small fist pump. The clip and the blood flow were critical, and the report was good. The doctors came out of the procedure pleased. There were no complications, and Holly left the room smiling and teasing me.

As Holly left the procedure room, I called out to her, "Hey, sweetheart. How's it going?"

She turned and smiled at me and said, "Who are you?"

When I finally left the hospital today around 8:15 or so, I was an emotional wreck. As Holly settled in after the procedure, she was very, very confused. This is a symptom of the vasospasms. How much of a cause for concern...who knows? Staff was aware and felt it was expected. How do the spasms transition to stroke? What are we looking for? What are we monitoring? It's all being checked. I have been unable from the start to Google or research anything. Just too terrified. I am at total peace with trusting the doctors 100 percent. They have been and continue to be great. Sharley is back in Massachusetts but continues to be my support. She is truly amazing.

Once again, trying to end on a good note. Earlier today, Holly had her first occupational therapy visit and wanted to show off. She got a few questions wrong but when being tested on what she felt, she got more excited as the test went on. First...

"Where am I touching?" the therapist asked.

"Left thigh," Holly said.

"Where am I touching now?"

"Upper right calf."

"OK, how about now?"

"You're making a diagonal left-right motion on my right forearm."

Needless to say, the therapist was pretty amazed. Holly, not missing the opportunity to show off on a test, dazzled the therapist four days after undergoing six hours of brain surgery with major complications.

This is our world these days. Highs and lows and madness. She makes me smile and cry daily as I watch her fight through this. I know that she's rocking anything she can control and fight through, and I suffer when she feels pain or confusion. It's hard to let go. It's just brutal. She was pretty confused when I left tonight, but today should, in the end, be viewed as a victory. Aneurysm is clipped tight, and blood flow is good. A collective fist pump is warranted, but now we hope the vasospasms remain as such, with no progression to something more serious.

As always, I do not reply to all e-mails or texts, but I read every one. They are my and Sharley's support. The socks and cards have begun to arrive. Please know during this critical time that I cannot thank you all directly as they arrive, but I will when this process nears its happy ending. Every motion these days feels like it's being done underwater. It takes five times as long as it should for the simplest functions, whether a phone call or a text or a thank-you. If an e-mail or text or call or package goes unacknowledged, please know it means the world to me, Shar, and most of all, Holly. Please know that every note, thought, or prayer will be acknowledged when this trying time is over, if not now.

Thanks and love.

Please Stay

11:22 p.m.
Shar texted me:
Just talked to her nurse.
She is fine—status quo.
She said some of her comments are inappropriate,
but she said this sometimes happens
and what they expect after major brain surgery.
She said as soon as she tells her Greg
will see her soon in the morning,
she starts chilling.
Nothing to worry about!
Xoxo

I replied:
Thank you so much.
Text me once more before bed, please.

Shar texted:
You want me to call again?

I replied:
If you don't feel it's necessary,
I will chill. Sorry.
It was just such a good day,
and then she got so loopy just
before I left.
If the nurse and you are OK, then so am I.

Shar texted:
I feel OK,
but why don't you call when you get home.
It will make you feel better to hear the info directly.
It's OK to double-check.
Whatever you need.

Karen e-mailed:
Greg,

Thank you again so much for keeping us all informed. Please, please, do not stress about responding to folks. We are all so grateful for all you are doing and feel nothing but love toward you both. I'll plan to come Thursday afternoon to give you a bit of a break, unless I hear otherwise from you, which is also totally fine. Whatever is best for you and Holly—me being there or not—is what I want to do. Even feel free to text on Thursday anytime and say never mind don't come or conversely ask me to come tomorrow or Friday or whatever. You and Holly are my top priorities. I get done teaching at 1:30 on Thursday and have borrowed a car so can drive out right after.

I replied to Karen:
Karen,

Holly is in a weird state with the vasospasms and just her brain healing in general. It should work, and I am so grateful, but let's chat tomorrow. Call me when you have a moment, and I will ring you back.

Karen responded:
Yes, definitely. Whatever works. I'll call tomorrow.

12:29 a.m.
Shar texted me:
Do you want me to call again?

                                                                I replied:
                                                                 Just rang.
                                                        Nurse in with her.
                                                  Calling again in ten.
                                                   Will text you after.

Please Stay

Shar texted:
OK!
How was dinner with Maura?

I replied:
Dan was good.
I think he had only low expectations about Holly's condition.
Maura was a bit concerned,
as Holly talked a whole lot of nonsense when they saw her—
truly out-of-character, vulgar things.
It was pretty wild and disconcerting,
even for me.
Maura, seeing her for the first time,
was really upset and can't understand how
Holly's brain is functioning.
Text you in a few, once I talk with her nurse.

Shar texted:
K!

I replied:
Just called.
All good at hospital.

Shar texted:
Having my second dinner now—lol.
Hol would be proud of my appetite!
I am off 2mro from work.
Pls let me know what I can do!

I replied:
All good.
Time for bed.
Call or text you in a.m.

Shar texted:
Indeed!

Keely e-mailed:

Oh, Greg!

Today was a good day, for sure. I know they are all *hard*, but this day sounds good. Angiogram *done*. *Clip* is good. Holly is excelling at tests!

You are doing great! I know you have to be *exhausted* in a way none of us ever knew was possible. I am amazed by you and Holly both.

Love love love and you never have to reply or call me.

Marjorie e-mailed:

Greg,

A big fist pump coming your way! Much love.

She is so amazing, and you are an absolute rock star.

Inge e-mailed:

Dear Holly and Greg,

I have been reading your updates with bated breath every day and am thrilled to hear about your daily triumphs!

Various churches all around Paris now have candles burning for you, as I make a stop on my daily wanderings to send you both a little flame of love and prayers. Yesterday it was Saint Clothilde in the ritzy seventh arrondissement. I've got you covered here!

The angiogram result was certainly a big hurdle cleared, but I left the hospital that evening more than a bit confused. Holly, after having made great strides over the previous few days, had regressed suddenly that evening. She greeted some dear friends with a string of curses and a coarse joke, most of which made little or no sense. Her friends found it scary and disconcerting, as did I, though the nurses said not to worry. Holly's friends had yet to see her prior to that visit and were relying on my reports on how well she was doing in the days leading up to their time with her. I couldn't help but think as we went to dinner that our friends thought I was putting an incredibly positive spin on Holly's progress. Maybe they thought I was in denial and that she may never be "Holly" again, which would be understandable after a grade 4 brain bleed. The short twenty-minute interaction between Holly and our two close friends that evening really hit me hard. I was drained. While I had seen her do well over the previous few days, maybe there would be a new normal—one that I could not conceive (nor did I want to).

DAY 10 — TIRED
April 30, 2014

Jim G. e-mailed:
Greg,
   You and her sister are showing incredible strength and fortitude. My mother had a brain operation for a very different issue and at one point suffered hospital psychosis, which finally passed. Look back a week and see how far she's progressed. It's a roller coaster for sure, but you are riding a few more downhills and less uphills. Godspeed to all of you. Everyone has your back covered here.

I replied to Jim:
   Thanks. Will be coming into office, barring anything drastic, on Friday. Will be good for me to get out of hospital and see friends. We are on day ten, and I am broken down.

Jim G. responded:
I went through that when my mom was in the hospital for two weeks—you have to make a bit of a break, as hard as it is to do. She's got a plethora of care. It's OK for you catch your breath.

Annie e-mailed:
Greg,
   Holly is just amazing and fighting hard. She might appreciate a pedicure this week. Bright green is a good color for spring and "rebirth." :-)

Kiss for Holly (one for each little piggy) and a hug for you. Stay strong for her and get enuf sleep!

Kerry e-mailed:
Morning, Greg:

I read this just now and have to say this is a true testament to your strength, although it sounds like you feel you don't have any. Holly definitely does, as all your e-mails have made clear to me. I am a bystander, but if you need anything, please do let me know, and I hope this message will give you more strength for today and tomorrow and the day after that. And rest assured, I have read every one of your e-mails but have not replied to every one because they are very humbling to read, and I cannot imagine what it is like to go thru something like this. As I told you, my daughter went thru surgeries when she was a baby, and I felt completely helpless and pretty numb. She got thru them all and is now giving me a run for my money. Holly will do the same for you, and, well, she already is! One day at a time, but you know this, I am sure. Just know too that you are not alone. You and she are in my thoughts and in my prayers and will continue to be.

8:52 a.m.
Shar texted me:
Morning.

I replied:
They are checking on her now.

Shar texted:
Who?

I replied:
ICU doc, and others making rounds.

Shar texted:
Oh great! Was confused.

I replied:
I am really struggling today.
But Holly's neuro signs and strength still good.

Shar texted:
Are you tired or sad?

I replied:
Both.
Holly's pretty confused
but not as bad as last night.

Shar texted:
If you decide to work Fri,
I promise you will feel better after that.

Dorinda e-mailed:
Greg,

Such good news. She is one of the strongest-minded women I have ever met! I knew from the beginning that she, of all people, would make it through this! She is an amazing girl. Her love of knowledge and life is like no other. She will pull through this. She's lucky to have you by her side.

Love you.

Still praying! And will continue…

Elizabeth e-mailed:
Greg,

Thanks for the update, my sweet friend. You certainly have a gift for communicating this journey. That's impressive in itself!

You just hang in there and go for the ride, though I know it's like the scariest roller coaster of all time. I have faith in you, and I am proud of you.

Please Stay

3:13 p.m.
I texted Shar:
Cynthia just left.
Holly talked to her for four straight hours.
I just left room.
She's got a small fever,
and I want her to rest.
If anyone comes in to her room,
she will talk and talk and talk.

Shar replied:
Cynthia must have loved chatting!
We went thru this last Sat.
Good job leaving. Ru home?

I texted:
New nurse.
She's watching Holly pretty carefully
because she keeps trying to untie her restraints
and leave.
Everyone laughs at her, particularly
When she says, "Just a second.
Untie me for a second.
I'll be good, I promise. Just untie me."
Everyone just smiles and shakes their head no.
Holly asked about eighty times today if she could leave.
I may try to bail around 6:30
to have dinner with Tommy and his wife.

Shar replied:
No prob at all.
New nurse is good, very attentive.
Please go out with Tommy.
I will call as many times as you like.

It will do you a world of good.

Xoxo.

Keri e-mailed:
Hi Greg,

I haven't contacted you in fear you have been and are being overwhelmed with a ton of questions and requests for updates on Holly.

My brother Richie and Shar have kept me in the loop, so I have been keeping up.

I do, however, want you to know that I am thinking about you guys daily and keeping both of you in my prayers! If there is anything I can do in Texas, please don't hesitate to contact me.

Give her a big hug from me, and let her know I love her very much!

From: Payan, Gregory
Sent: Wednesday, April 30, 2014, 10:12 p.m.
Subject: Holly Wednesday Update

Thank you all again for my evening group-therapy session and for allowing me to update everyone after a few glasses of wine this eve. Went to dinner with two dear friends tonight, trying to normalize for just a few, and when leaving, we spoke about the fairly well-known quote (forgive me if I don't get it verbatim), "To the world, you may be one person, but to one person, you may be the world." And it really is true in instances like this.

You cannot imagine the difficulties in performing everyday functions when every ounce of your being is directed toward another person.

Why can't you get off the couch? Because all you think about is a good day for someone you love and not rolling over and starting the day.

Why does it take twenty minutes for a three-minute shower? Because you are thinking, "Please let her not get a headache today."

Why did you fall over when putting your pants on? Because all you care about is a doctor saying, "She's doing OK," after a three-minute neurological exam. You don't care about simple everyday functions to prepare yourself for the day. Every minute of every day is focused on someone outside of yourself. You cannot read, eat, or sleep, because you don't give any thought to any function you would perform for yourself in a normal environment or existence. That is what it's like to go through something like this.

Based on how harrowing the last week and a half has been, I am optimistic in saying it was a good day. With no procedures planned, Holly was just supposed to be. Be a patient in a hospital ICU, eating bad hospital food, all while trying to get through another day of fighting vasospasms. She had a physical-therapy appointment that went great. They would have walked her today, but she has very high blood pressure right now. It's being kept there medically to combat the vasospasms. All other exercise and mobility was great, according to the therapist.

Holly chatted all day long. The biggest issue we had with her is that she's restless and will not, under any circumstances, sit still. She must have asked me seventy or eighty times to cut her restraints so we can either 1) get dinner, 2) take a bath, or 3) work on lesson plans. It was a bit frustrating, but she was asking nicely, for the most part.

She is still very confused by the spasms and is still seeing some things she shouldn't in hallucinations. But she's not in any major pain, and she ate and drank well today for the first time in ten days. A bit of a fever was noticed in the afternoon (101.4), and they blamed that for a bit of her confusion as well.

She started the day very well but noticeably tailed off. She really did need rest, but much like the last time she did this (the first day her breathing tube was out), she was full of energy. She was a lot crazy, a little frustrated, but warm and funny for much of the day.

Please know that absolutely nothing is being done for her brain rehab yet. That is all to come later. Right now, we are to engage her without overstimulating her, always bringing her back to the present by asking lots of questions about friends, family, life, and trips. The ICU's job is solely to keep her alive through the twenty-one-day window after the bleed. We are told regularly not to worry about the confusion and the hallucinations. That is all expected, particularly in this window of time after the bleed, and just six days after major brain surgery that had complications. She should be viewed as doing good.

Today's funny Holly-ism: A small group of doctors were in the room when Holly was being evaluated this morn neurologically. (By the way, she did great.) She took the opportunity to show off, as she usually does. When asked if she knew what building she was in, she said, "Some type of colonial, I believe."

When told it was a hospital and why was she there, she replied with a smile, "It has come to my attention that I'm having difficulty performing normal cognitive functions." Again, with a smile.

Then, when asked to count backward from ten, it was not good enough to go to zero. She went through to negative numbers.

It was quite a performance, and it drew smiles from the staff. Throughout the most difficult time of her life, she is bringing smiles to others and fighting with every ounce of her being.

I think she's doing really well, under the circumstances, while also being very, very confused as she goes through the vasospasm period. It's nasty and not pleasant, and she certainly says some things totally nonsensical and off-the-wall. But if you spend even just a bit of time with her, you recognize her as totally the woman we know and love, with her observations and sense of humor. It's a little scary but also a little encouraging. She's in there, undoubtedly, as we know her. I have not been prone to hyperbole through this, but I really, truly believe that I have seen enough to know that if she clears the twenty-one days after the bleed, she will make it back. There are just too many signs that make you smile and know that it's all in there, if not totally connected just yet, as the clinical signs obscure her ability to think fully just a short time after her surgery.

Many things still to work through over next ten days (heart issue, stunned myocardia; vasospasms; possible stroke; ICU psychosis; the drain in her head; the wound; and so on), but there is a hint of optimism in the air today, and I go to bed with just a tiny bit less stress than yesterday…

Thanks and love.

10:10 p.m.
Shar texted me:
Just picked up purple nail polish
for Holly to make her toes pretty Friday
when I come back.
I think purple toenails will make her happy.
Xo

Megan e-mailed:
Greg.

Thank you. Every night, I sit in my kids' room and wait for them to fall asleep and for you to send your update. Then I can think about going to bed. This is so hard, and you are IT—you are the world, and she is yours. There is no parental backup for her, and that is huge. So thank you for saving Holly when she started this horrible journey and for staying strong and keeping us in the loop. There are so many people who love and adore Holly, but you're the only one that can do what you're doing.

When Holly was here in September, Connor was singing this song on his seesaw: "Seesaw, Margery Daw, Jack shall have a new master; Jack shall earn but a penny a day because he can't work any faster." She found it to be hilariously inappropriate with themes of child labor, etc., and since Connor sings it often (too often), I get a little kick out of remembering Holly's reaction every single time. It helps me. :)

Tanya e-mailed:
Greg,

We are grateful at Drew as always for your passionate, vulnerable, and insightful updates about Holly—and you. I'm glad to hear that you had some time with friends tonight for refreshment and renewal. It takes a lot of energy to be the caretaker. We are in prayer for thanksgiving for what has been and in prayer for hope for what is to come. Peace and blessings. Sleep well.

<u>11:49 p.m.</u>
I texted Shar:
Just called hospital.
Holly well and sleeping.
Fever back, and she's getting Tylenol.
She talked with her nurse about Costa Rica.
All is well.
Good night. Xoxox

Erin e-mailed:
Hey, Holly.

Erin here. I'm the spunky, opinionated character from tenth-grade English and creative writing. Thank you for teaching us all of those vocabulary words.

Please Stay

I especially loved getting to draw them, even though my art skills never surpassed stick figures. And thank you for introducing me to the greatness that is Sandra Cisneros. Her brightly colored house will always be inspirational to me. Thank you too for your elaborate explanation and context for the *Iliad*. And thank you for coming to my college graduation. I'm pretty sure you had to sacrifice a rare and valuable free Friday night to watch me walk the stage. And thank you for opening your classroom to me so that I could learn from the best teacher (that's you!) how to be a good teacher. I really try to make you proud.

I told you a thousand times, but you're kind of my hero. Like, so much my hero that I have a picture of you and me sitting on my bookshelf in the living room. You have been instrumental in shaping my desire to become a teacher. In fact, it's no exaggeration to tell you that I don't know whether I would have graduated high school had it not been for your classes. For the first several years I taught, whenever I was confronted with something that was too complicated or too overwhelming for me to figure out, I would ask myself, what would Holly do? Just trying to think of what you would do—you with your infinite grace and kindness and positivity and hopeful outlook—usually guided me toward the appropriate action.

I also really appreciate that you introduced me to feminist theory and thought. Considering power struggles and the perspectives of those who are oppressed has given me a great amount of insight and empathy. I still tell people one of your quotable quotes: you told me that homophobes who justified their beliefs with the Bible were ignorant, because Jesus was always on the side of the oppressed. He rooted for the underdog, I think you said. I remember how revolutionary that thought was, although I'm sure that you conveyed it in a more eloquent manner.

I'm so grateful that we were able to meet in New York in December for dinner. I really enjoyed our chat. I left feeling so inspired. We both have big plans. So when you feel strong enough, wake up so we can get back to achieving them. I plan to see you soon. Maybe I can make it up to West Virginia soon. It's beautiful this time of year. I love you. Stay strong.

Greg Payan

Greg—thank you for being her best friend and her rock. It certainly means a lot to all of her friends around the world that you are able to be there with her. I know how much the two of you love and respect one another. If there is anything I can do to help you, please let me know. I am very good at ordering pizza and taking people to the airport.

DAY 11—SLEEPING IN MY OWN BED
May 1, 2014

I HAD SPENT TEN DAYS sleeping on my parents' couch at their home on Long Island. They were taking great care of me. Every night I would return from the hospital feeling a massive combination of brain fog and fatigue. I would walk in; drop my bag on the floor; and fall into one of their recliners, turning on the TV to distract myself from the day's events. My mother, upon hearing me enter, would pour me a glass of wine, ask how Holly was, and then make me dinner, regardless of when I came home and whether she was already in bed. It was wonderful having someone take care of me as I tried to take care of Holly, but after ten nights, I needed some normalcy in my life. I wanted to sleep in my own bed, wake up, and make breakfast in my own home. I wanted to take a shower in my bathroom and get dressed and go to work just as if it were any other day. I needed to go to work to see friends and colleagues who had been supporting me from afar while I devoted all my physical and emotional energy to Holly and what had transpired.

I decided I would return home that night and go to work on Friday. I planned to have dinner in my living room, sit on my couch, and watch some TV. I would read my mail, pay some bills, and try to pretend a little that things were normal, even though I would be kidding myself. Maybe I'd be better for trying.

6:37 a.m.
Shar texted me:
Sorry about not being able to get the report.
Just called this morning.
Spoke with her nurse.
The night went good.

Greg Payan

Holly slept for a few hours,
and she was less restless,
and they actually decided to taper off
one of the blood pressure meds.
so instead of trying to keep her BP over 140,
they try to keep it a bit lower
as they think vasospasm risk is lessening.
Love you.

           I replied:
           Thanks and talk later.

Shar texted:
Any extra help planned for today?
I feel like a bus ran over me,
and I'm not even there.
Pls take care of yourself.
Can I call for a massage reservation?
for you tomorrow or Saturday?

           I replied:
           As of now, I can barely move.
           I think I will make a reservation
           for a massage for Saturday.
           My plan is go to my place tonight and work tomorrow.
           My parents will be at the hospital tomorrow a.m.
           until you arrive.

Shar texted:
OK.
My massage was amazing.
Yes. Work plan for you is excellent!
You will feel really good, I promise.

           I replied:
           OK.
           Will make massage reservation online now.

Please Stay

Shar texted:
They usually say to schedule it later in day
and doing little after it's over is best for body,
I am at your disposal all weekend once I come back,
starting Fri around 12:30 p.m.

8:11 a.m.
I texted Shar:
She's resting this morn.
Out cold.
Nurse said she slept well too.
Taking another vasospasm test today.

Shar replied:
Glad she is resting.
Sorry about vasospasms.

I texted:
Maybe the numbers will be better today.
She's at the far end of the window of concern
where the risk should be lessening.

Shar replied:
Let's hope.

Guy e-mailed:
Greg,

Every day will bring something new. Be patient and embrace every moment. Holly will get through this.

Amber e-mailed:
Hi Greg,

My name is Amber, and I have been friends with Holly since seventh grade. I have always known Holly was an amazing person and friend. It's been a true gift to be able to call her a friend. Keely has been forwarding me the daily e-mails. I just wanted to write a quick note to say thank you for keeping us up to speed on Holly's progress. I can't even imagine how hard this has been on you and the entire family. I am so glad you are there with Holly and Shar. Shar is amazing too!

I just wanted to let you know that both myself and my daughter Ashlyn (ten years old) are sending positive thoughts and prayers up to Long Island from Maryland to you guys.

2:00 p.m.
Shar texted:
I am glad you are going home to your own place.
You will love having your bed for a night!

I replied:
Got the healing music going for Holly on iPad.
Karuna, her nurse, likes it.
Hol's got another fever though.

Shar texted:
Cool for music!
What is temp?

I replied:
Not sure.
They just said "a little fever."
Just gave her liquid Tylenol.

Shar texted:
Ask number when you can.
Just curious. How are delusions?
Did she get PT today?

I replied:
She's sleeping now.
She was trying to use bedpan earlier, and I left room.
Not sure if she was successful.
She's been a bit weepy this afternoon
as she has the skullcap back on for monitoring.

No PT today, I don't think.
I was sent out many times today,
so I may have missed it.
I am solo.

Shar texted:
Sad she's been weepy.

I replied:
She was in pain,
but I think some of it was frustration.
Was not as bad as Tuesday waiting for angio.
She's been in a bed for eleven days.
Talked with social worker about rehab facilities.
Will call and update you later.

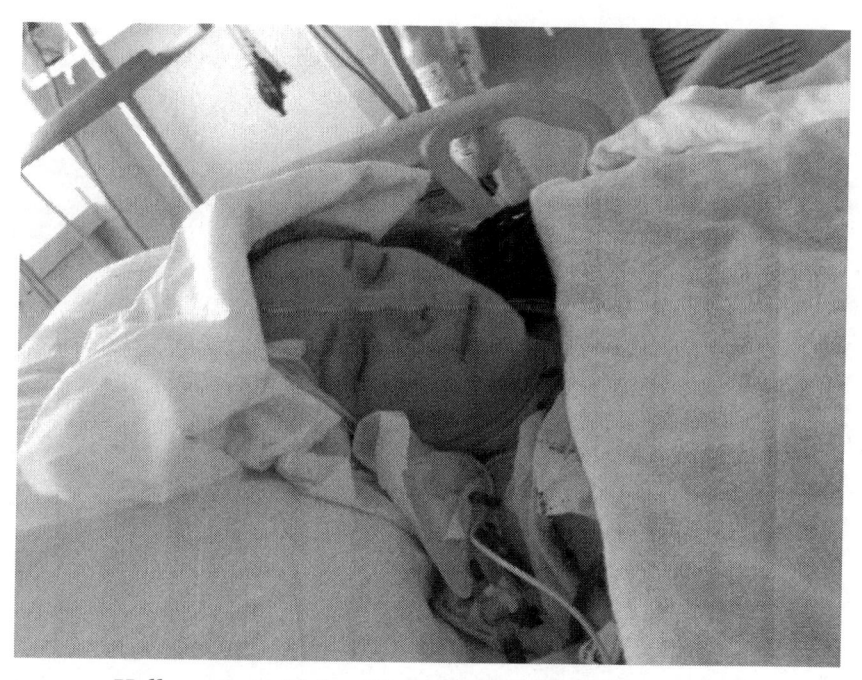

Holly resting with her "ice turban," a bag of ice wrapped in a pillowcase and placed around her head.

Brooke e-mailed:
Hi,
    I don't know if you were able to locate Holly's Spotify playlists. If not, here are some songs that I know she loves and a few I think she will:

1. "Song for Zula," Phosphorescent
2. "Doses and Mimosas," Cherub
3. "Sunlight," Bag Raiders
4. "Emmylou," First Aid Kit
5. "Closer," Tegan and Sara
6. "Shake," The Head and the Heart
7. "Elevate," Saint Lucia
8. "Don't Save Me," Haim
9. "All I Know," Washed Out
10. "Crazy," Au Revoir Simone
11. "Hanuman Baba," (Dub Farm Remix) Krishna Das

<u>**7:57 p.m.**</u>
Shar texted me:
Just spoke with nurse.
She's got a headache again,
so getting some orders for IV Tylenol.
They took catheter out earlier,
but she's retaining her urine and not releasing it,
so she will have to "straight catheter" her,
which means she just inserts temporary
tube and removes the urine.
It's a little bit uncomfortable,
but they're happy to have the catheter out.
Fever is gone.
Her nurse also said Holly did tell her
she had a brain injury and said,
"That's why I'm here."

Please Stay

> **I replied:**
> OK.
> Sad she's uncomfortable,
> but a mostly positive report.
> The rest is just making sure she's not alone
> and we're coming tomorrow.

Shar texted:
Oh yes.
How was your dinner?

> **I replied:**
> Pizza.
> Nothing special.
> Just good to be at my place.

Shar texted:
I bet.
Ur gonna have a great day tomorrow seeing work friends.
You just take it easy,
and I'll see you tomorrow night.

From: Payan, Gregory
Sent: Thursday, May 1, 2014, 8:08 p.m.
Subject: Holly Thursday Update

Two straight days with no complications and time to heal. Slight fever today and some head pain, as she had a sleeve on her head to monitor her brain waves and potential for seizures. She really hates it, and they can't give her much pain medication because it affects the test. Times like this, you just hold her hand and talk her through it, and it's just so hard. She's also a bit weepy, as it's really getting to her after eleven days in the ICU. Only halfway home, and she's just out of her mind. Uncomfortable, confused, and miserable.

Talked to a social worker today and even got a list of rehab facilities that Sharley and I will be evaluating over the next few days. I think that is the best sign we've had since she arrived. Vasospasms should start to get less by Monday, so that can't come soon enough. Tons of stuff still to monitor and work through, but if they are talking about next steps once she's released, I can't help but smile a little.

Tanya e-mailed:
Greg,

I continue to be grateful for your spirit, humor, and intellectual advocacy for Holly.

We are in prayer and thought here at Drew—both for you and for Holly and her family.

Thank you for giving us these updates on what are next steps and developments.

You are a gift—to Holly and to us. Peace.

Keely e-mailed:
Dear Greg,

Rehab facilities. Well, it sounds like y'all are working on hatching a plan to get out of that place, which is what Holly was ready for last Saturday! So it is for sure reason to smile!

ICU for eleven days with little to no pain meds would make anyone weepy. Just the past eleven days y'all have been through actually would make most people weepy, especially without drugs!

I (like everyone) can't wait for those stupid f'n vasospasms to be a part of the past. It's crazy b/c a week and a half ago, I'd never even heard that word before, but now it's a big cause of worry all day.

I hope you are able to get some good rest tonight. If you think of it, please tell Holly I love her and will be there within a day of her asking me to be.

I replied to Keely:
We will need you once she goes to rehab or just after. I think she's going to be a confused mess until she gets out. Once in the rehab facility, I think she'll take off like a rocket. Either once in rehab, or I think the best time is once she is out and on her own. We will see. But Holly is gonna need you. Just figuring out when.

Thanks and love love love.

Keely responded:
I am ready to be needed. Thanks for writing me back!

9:59 p.m.
I texted Shar:
I am *not* going to make it to 10:30 for the call.
I am in bed now and exhausted.

Shar replied:
No worries.
I will either call tonight or before work in a.m.
I liked report at eight. Good night.

I texted:
OK. Gn.

Some doctors and nurses would come by daily, reiterating over and over a version of "Just give it time. She's healing. She'll continue to get better." Others, however, would come by and stress the importance of being strong. Those doctors would say, "Things will be different. You just have to accept the new 'normal' once you're out of the hospital." Such statements were vague and also terrifying.

Would I be a caregiver and to what extent? Would I no longer be a partner? Being Holly's partner meant everything to me. Would I lose my identity as a partner in an equal relationship, and what circumstance required I become be something that could still give me fulfillment?

There were still complications to deal with. Not simple ones either. If we did get out and try to resume our old lives, what would life look like post-rehab? What changes would we have to make with our work? What changes would happen with us? What changes would occur with the lives we were living, which were working so well, and the lives we hoped to live together? I wanted to know what they looked like and if we could potentially still find happiness with Holly compromised intellectually and/or emotionally, but it was impossible to project out. No one knew...

DAY 12 — BACK TO THE OFFICE
May 2, 2014

6:46 a.m.
I texted Shar:
Checked in.
She's off one of the blood pressure meds,
but they did have to put the catheter back,
as she was holding too much urine.
Still no bowel movement.
Just stronger laxatives planned.
Some liquid Tylenol for a headache due to the sleeve.
She had an OK night. Mostly slept.

Shar replied:
OK. Thanks, G.
Don't worry;
they will get the bathroom stuff all worked out.
Her nurse told me last night it is all common
with what she has been thru.
Pls go to work and try to give your mind a little break.
I will let you know when I arrive and any pertinent info.
Xoxo

Mary e-mailed:
Greg,

Such good news that they are looking ahead! Been praying really hard! Tell her Cousin Mary sends lots and lots of love! And to Sharley too:) I can tell you are a wonderful man, and I can tell you truly love Holly! Makes me love you all the more and really look forward to meeting you one day! Thank you for the updates! They are much appreciated!

9:14 a.m.
Shar texted me:
Going five miles an hour in Greenwich
on the Merritt Parkway,
in case you wanted to let your parents
know why I am late.

                      I replied:
                               OK.
        At office, getting lots of hugs from colleagues.

Christy e-mailed me:
G,

You are being so ridiculously strong through this. Thank you for all you're doing for Holly and for keeping us up to date. I'm constantly thinking of her and worrying about her, but I also don't want to be a nuisance, so I am trying not to overwhelm you with e-mails/texts. :) That said, this weekend I am free on Saturday, so if you need anything, do let me know. I heard from Karen that Holly is not up for visitors (that totally makes sense to me—I think I would feel the same way), but if I can run an errand for you or take you out for a beer, or anything, just let me know. If not, I will continue to send positive thoughts to Holly (and you)!

  I replied to Christy:
  Yesterday she wasn't, but I had a visitor come in two days this week, and it went OK. Maybe next week, you or Karen can pop by. Trying to keep it just to her really close friends. More info this weekend when I speak with Sharley to check her schedule too.

Christy responded:
OK. Great. Just let me know, and I will be there. :)

11:45 a.m.
Shar texted me:
Just got here.
Will give you a report once I see her.
Walking in now.

I replied:
Thanks.

12:01 p.m.
I texted Shar:
How's it going?
I should be there around 5:30.

Shar replied:
OK.
Resting now.
She cried when she saw me
and then also began to cry
About other stuff.
Wants a board under her back or a new bed.
She told me she hates being here.
How is work?

I texted:
Was a nice distraction.
Holly's been a bit weepy last two days.
So that's been hard on me

Shar replied:
No problem.
Hope you embraced the hugs
from your work family.

I texted:
Let's talk more about rehab facilities when I arrive.
I want to talk to you and then staff.
Let's continue to play music whenever we can.
Is her head sleeve off?
It was making her insane.

Shar replied:
No, it's on.
Machine still going.
She wasn't complaining of that to me,
just how bad her back hurts
and why can't she move more.
She had me stretch and rub her legs.

Rachael e-mailed:
Greg,

My heart is absolutely breaking with this news, but I am so thankful that Holly has such a wonderful partner with her. I had dinner with you (and Holly) a few years ago here in New York and have lived vicariously online through y'all's wonderful adventures.

Holly was my English teacher and yoga (and life) mentor back in Texas in 2000 and remained a friend here in New York City when she first moved up to teach school in the Bronx. Holly is by *far* the most influential educator I had growing up. Of course, correct comma use and vocabulary words have been invaluable, but what she has taught me about resilience, peace, dedication, and patience are my daily go-to lessons.

The first couple years for me here in New York were pretty scary. I moved here for school when I was eighteen (with the help of a generous college recommendation letter from Holly), but I immediately lacked confidence in my decision to go to school so far away. I was home visiting family in Texas over Christmas and decided to stop by the high school to talk to Holly. She shared that she *also* was thinking of moving up to New York to teach at a school in the Bronx. She said she was scared about the change and wasn't sure if it was the right decision or not...even though it sounded exciting and appeared to be a great opportunity, she was still nervous.

In high school, I always looked up to Holly as this pillar of strength. Her inner core seems unshakable despite all of life's shit that has been given to her. So in that moment, it gave me so much comfort to hear that it's OK to be strong and also feel scared too. Those two can coexist. The strongest people are allowed to feel shaky, and maybe those moments are even what gives them their strength. It's such a simple "duh" thing to know. But it was a crucial aha moment for me as a scared nineteen-year-old who felt defined by and alone in my uncertainty. Even though I'm sure she doesn't know it, Holly gave me permission not to let those feelings of weakness define me. And I'm not sure I would still be here in New York if I hadn't learned that from her when I absolutely needed to in that moment.

I don't doubt that both Holly and you are feeling scared and weak in the most colossal way. So knowing Holly, it must just mean she'll come out of this an even stronger woman than before (if that's even possible). I have so much love for her (and for you), as everyone does, and will be using every ounce of that love to hope for a remarkable outcome tomorrow morning.

I replied:
Just want you to know that I relayed your story to Holly last eve before I left for the night, and she cried. She was very moved.

I plan on repeating it to her over and over throughout this process about being brave but scared. I think it's appropriate. Not scared for how this is going to turn out, but scared because a hospital is a scary place when you wake up there in restraints with machines and strange people and all else that goes along with it.

She's really going stir-crazy. But I will make sure she continues to be brave through the process.

Rachael responded:
Greg, thank you so much for passing on that story to Holly and for passing on her response to it. (I just put some silly socks in the mail today that Lauren and I picked out.)

I actually recently illustrated and wrote a children's story about this strength-through-sadness idea. I'm going to mail it your way as well. It's about a small lima bean that gets frustrated with his size. But even small lima beans cry big tears. And in the end, it's the self-watering from his tears that helps him sprout and grow tall. I've been imagining both you and Holly as lima beans, sprouting and growing, this week.

Your strength through this and absolute openness/honesty about your fears on this emotional journey have been inspiring. I appreciate your detailed updates (especially the funny Holly-isms you end with), as I am sure everyone does.

Obviously, I assume that everything is too overwhelming right now for visitors, but please let me know if/when any visitors would be welcomed/helpful/desired. Would still love to come out there if it would help Holly feel less stir-crazy for a bit.

<u>**5:51 p.m.**</u>
I texted Shar:
Bad traffic whole way.
There soon.

Shar replied:
No problem.
We are chilling. No bm yet.
Come on back when you are ready.

I texted:
Is she still tied?
I think she feels less crazy when not tied up.
It's a bit more normal.

Shar replied:
Her left arm on my side is tied, just loosely.
But yes, totally agree with you.
Wish she wouldn't tug at things so much when not tied though.

I texted:
Can you check on her Tylenol?

Shar replied:
Sure.

From: Payan, Gregory
Sent: Friday, May 2, 2014, 8:08 p.m.
Subject: Holly Friday Update

Another "good" day in Manhasset. It's all relative, but clinically Holly continues to do great. Sharley is back in town, so I am better. She is a confidant and friend, and she exudes strength and positivity, much like her sister. I am stronger when she is here. Plus, she's a wonderful dinner date after a long day. As her sister does, she brings me great joy.

Realistically, Holly's recall and other brain functions are of zero medical priority until she leaves the ICU and moves to rehab. That said, my feeling was that her lucidity today was the best it's been since the incident. While she was still confused, we had multiple conversations that could have taken place outside a hospital setting, including a long conversation about going to bed and finding a spiritual reason for enduring what she's going through. She is in terrible pain from a sleeve on her head that is measuring her brain function. It's tight and causing her great pain. In addition, she's been in a bed for eleven days, and her body aches beyond anything we can comprehend. She is miserable. Everything aches all over. She's confused by the alarms, beeps, fluorescent lights, restraints, leg compression sleeves, needles in her arms, and drain in her skull.

She woke up with all of this after falling asleep in her bed on a Sunday evening with me by her side, and she, along with many others who endure ICU psychosis, cannot comprehend what happened. My feeling is that until she can get out of the ICU, her confusion will remain. As time goes by, I do become more confident of how it will all come together once she does move to a rehab floor and then to a rehab facility. I have no doubt.

That said, she's still confused and in constant pain, with little relief from the Tylenol they provide her. Heavy painkillers are not an option because they can impair the monitoring of her neurological signs. That is the most important thing for the next ten days. It's horrible to say, but that is a priority over her day-to-day pain management, by my observation. They truly are trying to find a middle ground, but in the end, they need to be able to monitor her functions above all else. Hardcore pain medication would obscure that.

Holly is moving forward. I do feel really good about things, although it kills me to see her suffer. Visits consist of back rubs, foot rubs, hip rubs, arm massages, leg massages…you get the picture. Sharley and I try to engage her, but more important, just try to get her comfortable and aware.

The cards, socks, and other items have begun to arrive. The socks are selectively being used during her stay, but many of the cards and beautiful e-mails sent early in this ordeal will likely be shared when she is transferred to a rehab facility and when she can truly process them and they will give her strength. She will need it, and I think she will really feed off them. Please know that all thoughts, prayers, gifts, and such will be shared when the time is most conducive.

Know that with her spirit, strength, and intellect, I'd be shocked if, given the time and resources, she does not return to everything we know her to be—scholar, intellect, friend, traveler, dancer. Wonderful woman, brilliant, liberal, and kind. I have little doubt.

While going through a menu of the tomorrow's meal choices, I mentioned eggplant as an option. The nurse was present, and as I often do these days, I tried to ask questions when mentioning things. I said, "Sweetheart, what color is eggplant?"

She replied, "I think I'd say it's aubergine."

I said, "Is that blackish-purple?"

She said, "Oh, honey, you don't know?"

I said, "Are you embarrassed to be with someone who does not know what color aubergine is?"

And she said, "I'll let it pass."

She's doing well. She's improving. A change of venue is on the agenda, and only then will she truly be able to take the next steps she needs to take to get all the way back. Right now, the priorities are different, and the hospital staff totally know what they are doing.

Keep the thoughts and prayers coming. As she becomes a bit more lucid, she struggles more and more with the bed and all the other things that come with it. As all clinical signs move forward, it becomes harder and harder for her to comprehend lying in a hospital bed for eleven straight days with all the tubes, monitors, and everything else.

Thanks, as always, for keeping her in your thoughts.

Cynthia e-mailed:
Greg,

This e-mail really made me smile. I love that my aubergine-knowing friend continues on the up-and-up. Keep these e-mails coming. I keep worrying that you'll taper them down! We'll let you do that when she gets to rehab, but believe me, I wait all day to see these updates and am just thrilled to pieces with these last several days of very positive ones. Love to you, and give Holly a kiss.

P.S. Glad that Sharley is back. Let me (or Demy) know if you guys need some relief again. We are both more than happy to visit our sweet friend and give you guys a bit of a break.

11:49 p.m.
Shar texted me:
Just talked to nurse.
She's restless, trying to get comfortable,
a little confused.
Same story really.
She hardly ate.
I def think a chocolate croissant for her
in morning is a good idea!
Still just on one blood pressure med,
doing good with that.
Going to bed now. Xoxo

HH e-mailed:
Greg,

Thanks for the update today. I appreciate the level of detail you provide and can picture the exchanges. The aubergine story made me smile and does give hope. And hopefully with the upcoming transition, Holly will be able to find a little more relief in the situation…You were all in my thoughts all day.

I hope you are both finding some peace tonight and can rest.

DAY 13 — FEELING BETTER
May 3, 2014

~~~

The Friday I spent at the office gave me a huge emotional boost. I worked in an office in close proximity to my colleagues, many of whom I considered dear friends. I had spent countless hours with them over the years, both in and out of the office, accompanying many on work trips throughout the United States, Europe, and Asia. Seeing them and collecting hugs, kisses, and handshakes when they saw me for the first time since this all had happened was invaluable. In the coming weeks, I would try to get to the office whenever there was a window where coverage was arranged at the hospital through friends and family. It was a welcome distraction, and I always left feeling a bit better than when I arrived.

~~~

I e-mailed Demy and Cynthia:
What is your availability this week? I am really sorry to ask, but I am really exhausted and must try to start to return to work a little. I have my mom also, but if you can give me availability, it could likely help to just have you pop in for a few hours for a day or two.

Thanks so much. Let me know.

Demy replied to me:
Hi Greg,

Please—no apology necessary. That is what we are here for.

I am definitely free on Wednesday and can be there as early as you need, but I have to time it to be back in the city by three so I can teach. I can also rearrange my schedule to make it out on Friday. I can manage both days, if you need it. I can also do Tuesday after three, but not sure if you need evenings. On that note, I can do Thursday and Friday evenings too and next weekend.

I hope these times could work.

Elizabeth e-mailed:
Greg,

Thanks for the update, my friend. Like I've said before, your writing about this is so engaging and descriptive that it almost feels like I'm there with you in the hospital.

Holly couldn't have handpicked a better companion to help her through this journey, from the sounds of it. I am sure that sentence in itself is bittersweet right now, but I am sure her sister is *so* thankful to have you in Holly's corner, just as you are to have her in yours.

<u>8:35 a.m.</u>
I texted Shar:
She is sleeping, so I am in waiting room
They are making rounds.
I will bring the chocolate croissant in 15 when I go back.
She was OK on the overnight.
Just agitated.

Shar replied:
OK, thanks for update.
How ya feeling?

I texted:
Relatively good.
Sleeve off her head too, which is so good.

Shar replied:
Was just going to ask abt that!
Yay!
She must be thrilled!

Please Stay

I texted:
She's sleeping good.
Heart rate at sixty-eight.
Bp a bit higher but may be on purpose.

> **Shar replied:**
> Oh, good.
> What is bp—130/100?

I texted:
135/90

> **Shar replied:**
> That is OK, good #.
> They want her over 110 for top number
> to ward off the vasospasms!
> I prob won't be to hospital until 1:00, if OK?
> If you need me sooner,
> Let me know
> Xo

I texted:
We are fine.

> **Shar replied:**
> OK. I will check in around noon.
> Is she awake and talking more today?

I texted:
Yes.
She's doing great.
She now is having her chocolate croissant and coffee.

> **Shar replied:**
> How fantastic.
> Maybe the coffee will help her poop.

I texted:
Seriously.
Two weeks after a ruptured aneurysm,
and the biggest priority among staff
is seemingly that she has a bowel movement

Charlie e-mailed:
Greg,

    Thank you again for the update. Holly (and you and Holly's sister) have been in our constant prayers. We are so very glad that things seem to be moving in a positive, yet obviously cautious, manner. My family feels like, through your updates, they have gotten to know her, her pain, and her struggles. Although I know "difficult time" cannot begin to describe this ordeal, I think this "difficult time" has shown me another example of what true love should be. Know that *you*, as well as Holly, and your devotion to her, have been an example of love for all of us to view, and now live thru. God Bless…our prayers are with you.

Catherine e-mailed:
Greg,

    Hallelujah (really a "broken hallelujah," the L. Cohen [lyric] that a mendicant guitarist sang beautifully the Tuesday just after Holly's crisis began, when I was on subway on way to Drew. Kept me moving.)

    But the pain. I keep thinking of how you are practicing, because you must and you can, precisely what Holly means by "passionate nonattachment." [*This was the title of Holly's dissertation and soon-to-be published book*] Not exactly in relation to her, that doesn't resonate, but in relation to this necessary pain she is enduring. And you, with her.

Aaron e-mailed:
Hi Greg,

    Thanks again for the update. It sounds like she's improving by increments. It was great to see you yesterday. Thanks so much for stopping by the office. Hope you're able to get outside this weekend.

Aileen e-mailed:
Hey Greg,

    Glad to hear Holly is making progress. Sorry to hear that she is in so much pain. I can only imagine how awful it must be for her to go through and for you to sit by her side, watching her struggle.

It made me think that perhaps there are small ways to continue to ease her. Is it possible to get one of those eggshell mattress pads to put under her sheets? It might make a difference, and it helps with circulation.

For her muscles, can you maybe ask the doctors if it would be OK to use arnica or Yoga Balm? Yoga Balm works wonders, and I believe it is all natural. Maybe consider a heating pad or one of those aromatherapy pillows to place under her hips?

I don't know if any of these suggestions are helpful, but I wanted to just throw them out there in case there is something that can make her stay in ICU slightly more bearable.

I continue to look forward to your updates. You sound more positive every day.

12:52 p.m.
I texted Shar:
She's pretty tired now,
but she pooped—hooray!
Chocolate croissant and coffee worked magic.

Shar replied:
Hip hip hooray!

I texted:
A little bad news:
they are not getting a blood pressure reading
from her arterial line on the left side anymore,
so they need to insert one on other side.
Pretty big needle and uncomfortable,
as you know.
Grabbing lunch as they install new line.

Shar replied:
Oh man, sorry.
Just reading this.
Headed over now.
It is a beautiful day out!

1:51 p.m.
I texted Shar:
Outside on bench in sun now.
It's taking a little longer than they thought to put in the new line.

Shar replied:
The new line will be OK.
Don't worry.

I texted:
Xoxo

Kathryn e-mailed:
Hi Greg,

    Just want you to know that we continue to diligently follow Holly's progress here and are glad it continues to be mostly positive. I have sent a card and some socks today, so I'm sure they'll arrive early next week. In the meantime, hang in there—we are still sending wonderful love and good feelings yours and Holly's way.

Casey e-mailed:
Greg,

    Lots of love and prayers. Wanted you to see this from my friend Kinley, who only knows you through your words about Holly.

From:	Kinley
Date:	May 3, 2014, at 3:37:33 p.m. EDT
To:	C
Subject:	Re: Holly Thursday

I want to hug Greg. And Holly.

DAY 14—TOURING REHAB FACILITIES
May 4, 2014

From: Payan, Gregory
Sent: Sunday, May 4, 2014, 6:53 a.m.
Subject: Holly Sunday Update

Saturday was a bit of a roller coaster. Morning was great. Really great. She was sharp and starting to get why she was in the hospital, even saying, "You must have been really scared" when I described what happened two weeks ago. She started to cry a little. We kept talking. She still hasn't been eating too much. I asked the nurse if I could get her some coffee and a chocolate croissant, and she said that was fine. When I asked Holly if she wanted one, her eyes lit up. "Um…yeah!"

We talked a lot, and I was really, really happy for a few hours.

After her breakfast, they had to do a few things and noticed she had a problem in her A-line, which is a needle that goes directly into an artery to keep constant updates on her blood pressure. They had to move it to the other side, so now she's got needles on both sides, adding to her discomfort. Her head then began to hurt again, and she kind of regressed, getting a bit more confused and uncomfortable. While I can take a third Tylenol when I have a really bad headache, she just gets two. They continue to ration her pain medication, and again, she's just in a lot of pain.

Going to visit some rehab hospitals this morning, as Sharley will spend some time with her. Maybe I will be doing a bit better after seeing some light on the horizon. Doctors continue to tell me how great she's doing, and they know best. If everything goes perfect in the next eight days, she will be transferred out of ICU to another floor in the hospital to prepare for the transfer to a rehab facility, where I think we will see significant strides from the start. As I continue to say, as long as she's in a bed in the ICU, progress will be minimal.

9:26 a.m.
I texted Shar:
Just got to my first rehab place.
Going to two.
Took out the third on today's agenda,
as it was just too far out on the island.

Shar replied:
OK.

I texted:
Hope you're feeling better.
The administrator at the rehab place can't see me until ten,
so I am stuck for a bit.

Shar replied:
No problem. I am here with Hol.
Elliot is coming in to see her soon.
She is OK.
She had a CT scan earlier,
and they will look at prelim CT results
during rounds and discuss.

I texted:
OK. Thanks.
Real sad today about the reality of rehab.
Will make sure I get better before I arrive.

Shar replied:
It's OK.
I got really mad last night.

I will tell you abt it later.
She was in so much pain,
and they were offering her freakin' pill Tylenol!
I know they are taking such good care of her,
but I lost it.
Forgot to tell you, too,
nurse said they are looking at clamping head drain today—
not removing but just clamping off
to see if she maintains mental status
and they can evaluate to see if she can process fluid herself.

I texted:
Maybe we can speak to the doc after rounds
about different pain meds besides Tylenol.
Her pain is bothering me something awful too.

Shar replied:
Good luck on your tours!

Keely e-mailed:
Hi Greg,

The pain part is just real shitty! Sorry for my harsh language. But yeah, I mean, my gosh, if there's ever a time someone needs painkillers (and *more than* two Tylenol) it's after having brain surgery! Time just needs to hurry up and move along so y'all can move on out of the ICU.

It sounds like you are *both* doing remarkably well. It all has to be exhausting, but from my perspective, you are both superheroes. I'm worried about you with all the stress, so make sure you take care of yourself too.

Thanks as always for the e-mail!

10:44 a.m.
Shar texted me:
Elliot just came in and saw her.
She reached out for him to hug her,
and she started crying.
It was lovely.

I replied:
See if they can get her to walk too, please.
They keep pushing it another day.
Xoxoxo

Shar texted:
OK. I will find out.
Could you bring two bottles of seltzer for her?
She finished hers last night,
and I forgot to bring it today.

I replied:
Yep.
On way to second rehab spot now.
Call you later.

Shar texted:
OK. Physical and occupational therapy just came.
No walking today.
They did make her sit up and dangle her legs at the edge of bed.
Her head felt miserable sitting up,
so it wasn't long before she had to lie down again.
But she was upright, and that is HUGE!

I got back to the hospital after my rehab evaluation visits and sent Sharley back home to Massachusetts. The first three rehab places seemed OK, but I was not sold on any of the options just yet.

<u>7:15 p.m.</u>
Shar texted me:
Planning my yoga class for tomorrow night.
Breathe and get yourself outside once more.
It's beautiful!

Please Stay

I replied:
All good, thanks.
Have fun tonight.
Will check in before I sleep.

Shar texted:
K

I replied:
Last thing.
If Uncle Jimmy has a mushy pillow with feathers or little padding,
she needs one.
I will bring hers from home if he doesn't,
but since you're there in a.m.,
maybe you can try to bring one before I arrive.
She thinks her hospital pillow has too much padding.

From: Payan, Gregory
Sent: Sunday, May 4, 2014, 7:22 p.m.
Subject: Holly Sunday Update #2

Starting with the bad and always ending on the positive, Holly is beyond miserable being in her bed. If you sit next to her for an hour, she will ask a dozen times some variation of, "When are we leaving?"

She is not hallucinating anymore, which is good, but she cannot comprehend where she is and why, despite being told dozens of times a day. Her body aches all over, but if I had to guess, I think her head pain was a bit less today. I think it's just all connected, and she is just in a constant state of pain, more from lying in bed—although six hours of brain surgery surely did not help. I left a bit earlier than I wanted to today, mostly because I think she views me as her ticket out, and when I don't agree to facilitate that, she gets angry—at the world and at me. At various points today, she threatened to punch and kick me if I did not help her leave the room. However, in between, she extended her arms to the ceiling and said, "Come here."

I said, "What?"

She said, "Closer," and then she gave me a hug, as big a hug as she could. And when I left, we had a wonderful goodbye. I told her to be strong; she said she would and gave me a big kiss. When you step back and realize that the brain-injury patient is actually supporting the caregiver, if even for a moment, such awareness can cripple someone physically and emotionally.

OK, now the good clinical stuff. Doctors continue to say, Don't worry; she's doing great. Since her last angiogram, every test result has been positive. They also turned off her drain this morning to see if her body could process cerebrospinal fluid. The CT scan soon after, which checked the fluid and other brain stuff, looked good, and at the end of the day, her numbers on cranial pressure, a measure of her body's ability to process fluid, looked great. If this trend continues, it will be great news. She also did well at PT and OT this morning. She sat up in bed with her legs over the side. I was not there, but Sharley said that although she got dizzy very quickly, it was a good first step. Maybe tomorrow we can stand her up fully. Her neuro signs are good. She can push and pull with all her limbs, and her coordination seems fine. It's just that she is *soooo* weak. That is the problem, I think, with standing and walking as they dial back her BP meds. Hopefully, tomorrow she will stand and take a few steps.

There continues to be optimism about her condition. The mood has changed from *if* to *when* she gets out, and I checked out the first of a few rehab hospitals today. The clinical signs continue to be positive, but what she needs most of all is the mental and emotional strength for seven more days in bed. She really is at her breaking point and still has at least seven more days. Any strength you can send her way, she really needs it.

Thanks all.

It was an odd place to be in: instructed to search out rehab hospitals, where Holly would not be monitored 24-7. She was still on so many machines, and lots of scary numbers were still turning up as she battled vasospasms, which can sometimes be a deadly complication. I was scared to death.

I knew that once we were out of the ICU, her care would largely be my responsibility, even though she was being transitioned to an acute traumatic brain injury (TBI) facility first for an undetermined amount of time. I was hopeful about her prognosis, and I tried to be upbeat, but at that point, trying to imagine what our future life would be like dominated my thoughts. When I was alone at night, I kept trying to breathe, to relax, but more often than not, the quiet forced me to think.

I had heard rumors about restrictions on one's life after an aneurysm ruptures. Would Holly be able to fly and travel? Would she be able to surf? Would she be able to do yoga? Would she be able to drink some wine with dinner? Would she continue to have a career?

Holly is brilliant. She might still make a great life partner, and I was committed to her forever, but surely she'd have deficits of some kind. I hadn't done much research, but I had heard a few things, and the idea that she'd be able to return to her teaching job seemed incomprehensible after what she had been through.

About a week after her surgery, Holly had a conversation with a colleague and close friend who was in West Virginia and who desperately wanted to talk to her. I put Holly on speakerphone, as Holly was in restraints and could not yet hold a phone to her ear. The conversation was like the most awkward first date you can imagine, with two people speaking but yet not communicating. It was two minutes of awkward pauses and dead air. If she could not even have a conversation with her best friend, how would she teach a college class four months from now?

Were we insane to think she'd be returning to teaching so soon after what she had endured? Her career was a huge part of her identity. She had to make it back. And strangely, more often than not, I believed she would.

I often thought all those things I was panicking about meant nothing as long as I had her alive and healthy. But the more I thought about it—all those things were critical to her happiness. If she was going live a life without many of the things she loved, she would be absolutely miserable, and I would be too. Selfishly,

I wondered what my life would be like, living with someone who was desperately unhappy. What types of stress would this put on our relationship? There would have to be some modifications in our life, wouldn't there? Would our essentially charmed life fall apart? Only time would tell. I knew I had to hold it together, keep being strong, and continue taking care of her as best I could, so that time and circumstances would provide those answers.

DAY 15 — WINNING AN AWARD
May 5, 2014

8:05 a.m.
Shar texted me:
Morning.
I did call hospital last night around eleven,
but nurse was busy,
and I was asked to call back in thirty, and I fell asleep. :(
Packing up and heading over in a bit.

I replied:
OK.

Brian e-mailed:
Greg,
    Danielle and I read your update yesterday to the kids tonight @ dinner, and they all prayed for Holly. We also told them to offer any type of pain or discomfort they may encounter for Holly. We're really pulling for both of u to stay strong. You're both doing soooooooo great. I'm around all week, so I'd like to take u out for dinner—wherever u want and whatever day works for u. Doesn't have to be long or as long as u want. Just some good food and an ear that will listen. Let me know, buddy. Give Holly our love.

    I replied to Brian:
    Thanks for the offer. Slight chance Wednesday, but I am really buried. I have work, hospital, trips to rehab facilities for scouting them, and two photo shoots this week for NFL draft. I've kept

myself really busy to try and distract myself. If not Wednesday, maybe next weekend. Really appreciate the offer and the prayers. Will see how things shake out. Drop me a note Wednesday a.m. I can't keep track of life these days…

Brian responded:
U got it. Will speak on Wednesday. Try and get some rest, friend.

Dee e-mailed:
Greg,
   I can and imagine how hard it must be for her to be chained to the bed. And even more so for you to watch her struggle. I am here if I can do anything. I am happy to research and check out places. I know a few neuro psych people that might have recommendations.

Demy e-mailed:
Hi Greg,
   It sounds like it was a tough day—filled with great medical news, which is the hope. I know you are experiencing this whole situation the most compared to everyone (well, you and Shar)…Because Holly loves you and you are her person and she trusts you, you will get all the love, trust, and also the pleading and the punches. I am sorry that it is so hard! I am thinking of you and of Holly—and pray and have faith that she will find the strength to endure one more week. She has overcome so much. I will instill faith and hope in her as much as I can (and much much love) on Wednesday.
   I am sending much love and positivity and hope your way…Thanks as always for your amazingly detailed and genuine e-mails. I hope that you are taking care of yourself and that having Sharley back is giving you the strength and support you need.

10:09 a.m.
Shar texted me:
All is well.
Head drain still clamped and doing good.

They upped her Precedex (helped her relax last night).
She is resting now.
Lauren—thin, long brown hair—is her nurse today.
She was just trying to get Holly to eat,
but Hol said she wanted to rest some.
I have a latte and gooey pastry,
so I will force something down her
She's resting peacefully right now. It's nice to see.
Lauren said her night was fine.
I have a new pillow and will try it for her when she wakes up!
Xo

I replied:
OK. Thanks.
Have two appointments for more rehab tours Friday afternoon and will get appointments in Manhattan when I can.

Shar texted:
OK.

Jennifer e-mailed:
Greg & Sharley:

Thank you so much for keeping us posted on Holly's progress. You have all been in our thoughts and prayers...and how blessed Holly is to have you by her side!

I just put some socks in the mail for Holly and put together attached for photos to have in her hospital room.

Get Well Soon, Holly!

Your cousins all wish you a speedy recovery. Our wish is that you are "hopping and dancing" with us all again soon. We love you!

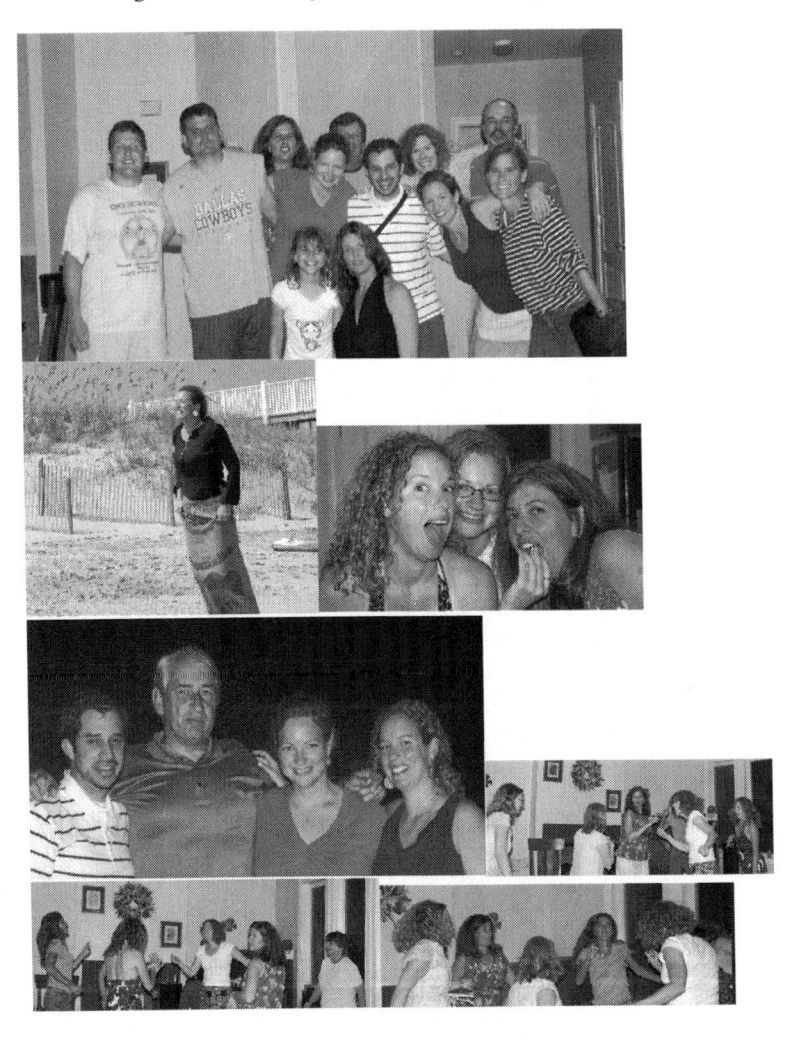

I replied to Jennifer:
Thank you so much, Jennifer.

We will get the printout done shortly and post it with the other photos in Holly's room. We're hanging in there as best we can. All the thoughts and prayers are greatly appreciated.

4:40 p.m.
Shar texted me:
I'm leaving now.
Karen is chilling with her.
Hol is good, resting.

I replied:
Great.
Have a safe trip home.
Am on train now and then heading over to hospital once I get my car.
Was she a bit better with pain and more sedation?
Did they try to stand her today?

Shar texted:
She was just resting most of the time I was there.
Nurse said it could be still from the meds last night,
or it could just be she didn't sleep so great.
No PT or OT before I left,
but they would only try to sit her up again.
She is too weak still to stand.

6:00 p.m.
Shar texted me:
Just texted Karen to see how it's going.

I replied:
OK

Shar texted:
Report from Karen....Holly's pretty well.
Had one moment of brief confusion (thought it was 2005) and loopiness.
But most of the day she was with it and having real conversations.
She's been sleeping a lot.
Had some pain when sitting up to eat.
They gave her Percocet.
The physical therapist came by.
Holly did well with in-bed exercises.
Was a bit too dizzy to sit up for long.
She had some blurry vision too.
She's uncomfortable but resting and hasn't been too confused.

6:52 p.m.
I texted Shar:
Got here a little while ago.
Just was with her for about half an hour with Karen.
Chatter the whole time.
Karen says she's so happy she came.
Holly is Holly,
and when the pain is not beating her down,
she's real lucid.

Shar replied:
Yay yay yay!
I am teaching yoga at seven.
I am dedicating my class to Hol and
will be reading about having hope in the present moment.
Xo.
Will check in with you after, around nine

Stephen e-mailed:
Dear Greg,
I don't believe you and I have ever met. I'm chair of the Graduate Division of Religion at Drew, and I've been relaying to the GDR faculty and students

the updates on Holly that Christy has been relaying to me. The expressions of concern, outpourings of love, and promises of prayers from so many quarters here in the Theological School have been immense.

This Wednesday evening at 6:30 p.m., we have our annual GDR Dean's Reception and Prize-Giving Ceremony. One of the prizes awarded is the Helen LePage and William Hale Chamberlain Prize. The prize description is as follows: "Established by Joan Chamberlain Engelsman G'77 and endowed in 2001 in her memory by her husband, Ralph G. Engelsman. Awarded annually for the PhD dissertation that is singularly distinguished by creative thought and excellent prose style."

Holly received a Pass with Distinction at her dissertation defense, as you probably know. Distinctions are granted rarely enough to make the recipient an automatic candidate for the Chamberlain Prize. The GDR faculty responsible for selecting the prizewinners decided some weeks ago that Holly's outstanding dissertation was the one most deserving of the Chamberlain Prize this year.

I'm only sorry that Holly will not be able to receive this honor in person. Please relay the news to her. Everyone at the ceremony will be thinking of her, even before the Chamberlain Prize winner is announced.

All good wishes to you and her as she continues on the slow but sure path to recovery.

I replied to Stephen:
Stephen,

Thank you for the note. I will relay to her when the time is right. I want her to be able to process it, and right now, while her neuro signs and intellect are great by all accounts, she is weak and still very confused. When she is out of the hospital and in a rehab facility, I will share the great news. Right now, her biggest problem is awareness of her situation. It's not uncommon for those who undergo a traumatic event followed by an extended ICU stay. She can have a clear conversation about things religion and teaching, but her environment is not something she can process yet. I am confident she will move forward by leaps and bounds upon her exit from the ICU. Thanks for the note, and please keep her in your prayers for strength and healing.

Stephen responded:
Thanks, Greg. I understand completely.
    Peace.

Herb (Holly's landlord in West Virginia) e-mailed:
Greg,
    We have been kept up-to-date via Brooke's e-mails to the college community. Several faculty members have been forwarding the messages. We were wondering about what we can do to keep things rolling. Would you like us to start the car every few weeks?

I replied to Herb:
Herb,
    As you can imagine, I am overwhelmed but promise to give you a call tomorrow or Wednesday at the latest. Trying to decompress for just a few right now.

Herb responded:
Sounds fine. Whenever you feel up to it.

From:	**Payan, Gregory**
Sent:	**Monday, May 5, 2014, 10:10 p.m.**
Subject:	**Holly Monday Update**

I think we can say it was a mostly good Monday. Holly remains very weak. She is still not able to stand and got very dizzy when brought to the edge of her bed to sit up. A little discouraging, but that will all come back in time as she continues to heal and

gain strength. She did not sleep much and was tired for much of the day, although when I arrived in the evening, she had a great first hour—lucid and asking lots of questions. One of her biggest problems is trying to understand where she is, why she's there, and why someone so brilliant is confused so often as she spends her days in the ICU on tubes and unable to sleep on her stomach (as she prefers) and in constant pain from her head to her toes. We explained it to her as best we could, and she really seemed to be getting it. Whether she gets it tomorrow has yet to be seen, but it was a really good night. She was lucid and really trying to pull it all together. She always has yearned for knowledge and awareness, and she's really trying to figure it out whenever she can.

She can still laugh, joke, and be sarcastic. She is playful and Holly in spite of her constant pain. I got a big hug hello, and we had lots of playful banter. When her hospital dinner arrived, I told her, "Honey, I put in a request for enchiladas *del norte* with extra mole sauce and a margarita, so I don't know what this is."

I got the exact reply I expected. She flipped me the bird with a smile. She even asked if she's gonna owe me big time when this is over.

I kissed her, smiled, and said, "Baby, if you only knew…"

Holly is in a lot of pain, and she's confused, but don't be mistaken. Her spirit and will are far from broken, and we are not allowed to be morose in her presence. When not in bad pain, she's very playful and likes to joke. We're even allowed to tease her, so I poke fun about her brain, which always brings forth a "Hey! No brain jokes!" from her.

If I had to guess, I'd say she slept really poorly last night and was real tired for most of today. I got a few good hours after arriving early evening, and when I left, she gave me the OK to go. I asked if she wanted me to leave so she could rest, and she said that was a good idea. I told her to look at me and said, "I want you to say, 'Got it,'" and she said yes. I told her to close her eyes and asked if she could still see me, and she said yes. Told her I was leaving and said good night as if I were putting her to sleep on any other night, but first she had to be able to see me when she closed her eyes, so she would not be scared after I left.

I'm still concerned that she's weak and not eating enough. I would love for her to stand, but she's just not up to it. I'd love for them to start giving her meds to fix her heart, which was damaged due to the incident, but they need to stabilize other things first. It's just going to take time.

When she's not too tired or in too much pain, her brain and neuro functions are great. She has come a long way. I was holding her hand during the nurse changeover tonight, and they went through her case. Normally, I avoid these like the plague, but I was stuck holding her hand as she rested. With five being the worst rating, her case had three fives and a four when describing her incidents. In spite of this, she can smile, joke, and tease and still knows the square root of thirty-six on command. I know you may be getting tired of my daily e-mails and incremental moves forward, but this is recovery from brain surgery. There are no one-day miracles—more like thirty- or sixty- or ninety-day ones. We are two weeks in from her initial bleed, which is nothing. She was not breathing when she arrived at the hospital. I'd love to say we spend our evenings reading *The New Yorker* together, but she's not there yet. She will be, and I'll be happy to tell you when she is. Please be confident that where she is right now after what she endured is nothing short of remarkable.

Thanks for everything. The love, prayers, and good thoughts across this group fuel me. Eventually the e-mails will slow, and if I miss a day, please don't assume the worst. It just means a new update will come soon.

Cynthia e-mailed:
Greg,

Thanks for the update. We are definitely *not* getting tired of your e-mails. I know the days must feel terribly long and the progress terribly slow, but your e-mails really do read to me like leaps and bounds of progress (intermixed with occasional but more minor setbacks). It may be hard to see it from the front line, but believe me, I get a sigh of relief each time I read one of your notes because things always seem a little better than the previous day, and that's what matters.

Thanks again for the daily updates and for all that you are doing on behalf of Holly. It means the world to me to know that she's got such a great caretaker/support/partner at her side.

HH e-mailed:
Greg,

Thank you for these. I wait for them every night. It's a great service you are doing for those of us who love her. Wishing you strength and peace.

Kerri e-mailed:
Hi Greg,

Thanks so much for the updates. I'm Shar and Holly's friend Kerri, from Arlington. Shar may have told you, but just in case she didn't, I mailed a package to you containing some nice dry shampoo. One is like a real powder in aerosol form. The other is more liquid. They both smell good, and I hope they are at least a little better than what they may be using at the hospital. I mailed it USPS, and it was supposedly going out today, so I have no idea how slow or fast it will get there. (Probably slow. Sometimes I think the postal service still employs ponies.)

About thirteen years ago, I used to cut Holly's hair. I went through hair school after college and have kept my license up-to-date in order to be able to keep getting salon-quality hair stuff for cheap prices. This may all seem like random info, but what I'm getting at is that if she needs anything related to hair care as she is being taken care of by y'all and the awesome hospital staff, just let me know. I'm happy to see if I can get good hair stuff to you for her. That's at the very bottom of the list of her needs right now, I know.

God bless you as you are walking through this with her. I'm praying for her and for you as well. Specifically, I'm praying that the weight of what you are dealing with will not feel like it is crushing you.

Thank you so much for your e-mails. I love hearing how you are both faring through this intense storm.

Blessings,

The Texan with hair products :)

Keely e-mailed:

Greg,

As always, thank you so much for taking time to write this e-mail…Y'all are on my mind so much that it feels weird that you weren't always on my mind. What did I used to think about?

I am sure it doesn't feel like it at all, but two weeks is not very long at all. I *know*—easy for me to say, sitting here watching the Lindsay Lohan docuseries on OWN (which, if you like borderline personality disorder cases, I suggest you watch)!

I'll work on things, Greg, but please keep writing and please know/feel you are appreciated/loved/supported/strong/amazing!

Ashley e-mailed:

Greg,

I'm so proud of you! You're doing great, and we should all be so lucky to have someone like you in our lives. Your strength and words are inspiring. The love, prayers, and warm thoughts are coming strong from Texas. She has lots of people who love her dearly. I forward your e-mails to my parents every night. She's been a part of our lives for so long, and they adore her too.

Stay strong and hang in there.

Erin e-mailed:
Greg,

I am a realist. Holly will be in the hospital for months. She is doing an extraordinary job rising to the obstacles that face her. However, I know that funding will become an issue. In that regard, I think I can help.

I hope that you will send me a message of support, as I am trying to organize a fund-raiser to be held concurrent with her birthday in July.

Here is what I envision: I have secured a space in a comic book store owned by her former student Matt. There will be a stage and a suggested donation for admission. We will have live bands, and my goal is to raise $5,000. I know this isn't much, but I hope that any amount will help. I plan to make this an annual fund-raiser and to continue it until her medical costs have been met.

All I need from you is a yes. Please tell me that I am right that funds will be a problem and that you would appreciate a fund-raiser.

I think it would buoy Holly's spirits to know all the people who are thinking of her, and I think it will not be difficult to find people to volunteer their time and energy to making some kind of effort that will improve her circumstances.

I replied to Erin:
Erin,

I think it's a great gesture. I have not yet spoken with her insurance company since the first day this happened but will today. Holly either has 80 percent or 100 percent catastrophic on her plan, according to her friend. There will be significant out-of-pocket expenses during her recovery, but I don't know if that will be five to ten thousand dollars or six figures plus.

Your gesture is wonderful. Thanks.

Erin responded:
Thank you for the support! I think people around here are eager to help. I know that a few thousand dollars won't go far, but I also know that every penny will help!

We'll move forward with planning!

11:48 p.m.
Shar texted me:
Just talked to her nurse.
She wanted me to tell you she really tried on the food,
but it was a no go.
Holly would not eat.
She was getting restless again,
and they upped her Precedex, I think she said.
She said once she started talking religion with her,
she calmed down.
everything else is status quo.
Good night, G!

I replied:
OK. Good night, Shar.
Rest well. She's in good hands.

DAY 16 — MORE VASOSPASMS

May 6, 2014

8:03 a.m.
I texted Shar:
Just saw Holly for a minute when I arrived.
She's being prepped for a CT scan.

Shar replied:
K.

12:01 p.m.
I texted Shar:
OK, I must leave soon.
Parents coming at three.
I will call you at two.

Shar replied:
OK!

Krista e-mailed:
Dear Greg,

Sending both you and Holly continued prayers for courage, stamina, and peace. I have not replied to your e-mails because I do not wish to overwhelm your in-box. But I am popping in quickly as a reminder that even people who are strangers to you (and only somewhat known to Holly) are holding you both in the light each and every day.

Soon I will send greetings (in the form of photos and socks) by mail.

Holly is herself a miracle to begin with. She is going to pull through. Wishing you strength and patience as you see her through. I hope you are finding ways to care for yourself too.

3:03 p.m.
I texted Shar:
More bad transcranial Doppler numbers and vasospasms.
They projected confidence though
and said it's way too early to get worried.
Issue identified, and they have it under control.
Ring you around eight.

Shar replied:
OK. No prob.
Hope to be at yoga.
Can call you
after.

I texted:
OK. Offer the class up for the three of us.
This is so hard. Xoxox

Shar replied:
Oh yes, of course! XO
It is going to be OK.
She is doing
great.

I texted:
We will talk later,
but doctors were so happy before that one TCD test.
Grrrrr.
Enjoy your practice.

Shar replied:
You working late?

I texted:
Yes.
Also, doctor who read the new scan was very calm.
Said, we see the issue. It's early.
We will treat it.

                                                        Shar replied:
                                                              OK. Thanks.

Dee e-mailed:
Holly,

    Once upon a time, four girls (by that I mean strong, independent, smart, and beautiful women) traveled to a far, faraway land. That land had beaches rather than concrete, thatched huts rather than skyscrapers, and surfboards rather than cars. That wonderful land was called Costa Rica—Pura Vida surf camp. I do not know if it was the magic of that place, fate, or coincidence that landed us all there on that particular magical week, but I do know that from the moment you were stung by the *agua mala*, I had met the most amazing friends of my life.

    Holly, I sit here at the beach in Montauk, listening to our wave, digging my toes in our sand, and thinking about how much I love you. I am thinking of your laugh and your smile. I am thinking about how you are so full of love that you give so freely to everyone in such a gracious and open way. Even to me when I least deserve it.

    OK, in all seriousness, I have learned so much from you: generous spirit, delicious food, how to have fun, how to really travel, and *dance parties*!

    The biggest way you showed me your love was when you took care of me through cancer. I was terrified, and everything moved so fast. You held my hand and went to the doctor's office with me to take notes, did yoga with me the day before my surgery. All of that with strength and compassion and grace. You took my fear from me when all the while I know it was the scariest thing for you to be managing cancer in your loved one after losing your mom and your husband to this terrible disease. I am grateful that you got me through it and gave me the courage to face it down, and more so knowing the courage you had to have to do it with me.

I think I could write all night of the wonders of you and all the things you bring to my life. You are the most amazing person I know. I love you so, so, so much. I know you are scared. I am scared too. I want you to know that I have learned to be courageous through these scary things and send nothing but love to you. I know exactly how to do that for you because I had the best teacher—you.

Love and kisses. I am not afraid of storms, for I am learning to sail my own ship.

7:34 p.m.
Shar texted me:
Didn't make it to yoga. In bed now.
I am OK not chatting unless you need to talk to me.

I replied:
Do you have five minutes?
My folks had a fun update.

8:39 p.m.
I texted Shar:
Just called, and you didn't answer.
My parents said their last hour with her was great.
Catheter removed. Holly used bedpan for first time.
She was laughing and joking and happy and ate like a champ.
Catheter still out.
They will see if she can use bedpan on overnight.
She was in a lot of pain this afternoon but is better.
She's still talking lots and seemingly fine
with the increased meds for the vasospasms.
My parents left and were excited to go back tomorrow
because they had so much fun with her.
Feel better yourself.
Talk tomorrow. XOXOX

Please Stay

After returning home the second time, Sharley really began to struggle. The emotional toll of trying to balance a critically ill sibling four hours away, her job, and her family began to manifest itself physically. Sharley just felt sick and not well enough to come back to New York. While I was terribly sad Sharley had begun to struggle, I could do nothing but love and support her from afar. She had sustained me to this point, and even though I was better with her beside me, I knew I could push through without her. She would not make it back to New York for the rest of Holly's ICU stay, and I was OK with that. She had done more than enough, and I just wanted her to get well and be there for her family.

On most days for the remainder of Holly's ICU stay, I would go to the office early in the morning and get to the hospital by midafternoon. Sometimes I flipped that schedule, depending on when my parents or Holly's friends were available to spend time with her.

From: Payan, Gregory
Sent: Tuesday, May 6, 2014, 9:24 p.m.
Subject: Holly Tuesday Update

A lot of ups and downs today. Wound up doing a morning shift at the hospital before heading to work. Had a great time with Holly, though she was a bit sleepy. We laughed and talked, and when the doctors did their rounds, she got all her questions right, and then said, "Give me something harder."

I asked her what the square root of sixty-four is, and she said, "Eight o'clock…I mean eight." And then she laughed.

The doctors asked me to step out of the room. They said she was doing great. They just wanted to check one thing, but they thought they could take the drain out today. One doctor went back in the room and said, "Holly, let's make a deal. You eat a good breakfast, and we'll take the drain out." And they shook on it.

I left as they did the one test they wanted to double-check. I was really walking on air and feeling so good about things. After arriving back in Queens to go to work, I got a call from the hospital. Her transcranial Doppler numbers were up for the second straight day (the double-check test), and they wanted to do another procedure to confirm. They did the procedure, and sure enough, she's still experiencing vasospasms. It's the only issue, seemingly, in her recovery, but it's a *huge* one. Vasospasms can lead to stroke or worse. I spoke with the attending doctor, and she assured me that they are noticing it early, they will treat it, and they will deal with it. I asked if I could exhale, and she said yes. It's not uncommon in patients who had the type and severity of her bleed. It's serious, but they know how to combat it. I did as I was told and tried to exhale and trust in the experts.

My parents did an afternoon shift and said the first few hours were difficult. Holly was sleepy and in a lot of pain. She was given liquid Tylenol and then Percocet. She kept wanting to get out of the hospital and to go to the bathroom. Finally, after hours of her asking to go to the bathroom, the nurse acquiesced and removed her catheter. Sure enough, Holly was able to go for the first time since arriving. After that, my parents said, her mood changed markedly.

She spent the last ninety minutes of my parents' visit talking, laughing, joking, and…eating. She ate two yogurts, ice cream, a spinach-and-cheese croissant, and a brownie. This, really, is about what she's eaten in a week before today. My parents were amazed, and I was too, listening to my parents relay this to me over the phone.

I don't know what to think. My parents said they are looking forward to going back tomorrow. They were actually having a good time when they left. The meds for the vasospasms likely will continue to give her headaches, but they are necessary. The doctors seem confident that they know the issue, and it's treatable. In a call later today, the head nurse confided that if she didn't have the vasospasms, they may have had her leave a few days early, in fact. Now that will not be the case, and she may even have added a few days on to her ICU stay. They are being conservative, and I am in total agreement.

I guess that in the end, up…down…then up again is a net gain for the day. I'd be lying if I said this wasn't making me insane though. I need to decompress for a bit before calling the night nurse for another update before I try to get a few hours of sleep.

Thoughts and prayers for Holly and any voodoo spells to ward off vasospasms also greatly appreciated.

Good night, all.

Kandrea e-mailed:
Hey, Greg.

Just short and sweet, but I wanted to let you know that you are an amazing man. I couldn't be happier that Holly has someone so strong and intelligent to be by her side. Thanks for all that you are doing for her. But please know that we are all here for you, and all of your families, just as much we are here for Holly.

Thank you for taking such amazing care of someone we all love so much. I know that it's not easy, but your strength and love give us all inspiration. Just like Holly, you are definitely added to my list of people to admire.

Keely e-mailed:
Greg!

F*ck those vasospasms! I don't know any voodoo, but I am ready to head to Louisiana and find someone who does!

I was trying to understand everything at this point. While she was still fighting potentially life-threatening complications, I was optimistic Holly had made it through the worst. We could spend time with her, talking and laughing, and often convince ourselves we were with the old Holly at times. At other times, she was not in any intellectual state where I could see her resuming the life of an academic.

In the ICU, we were asked to fill out Holly's meal requests a day in advance from a printed menu so they could custom-prepare meals for the patients. Earlier that afternoon, I was reading the choices to Holly, and she was totally unaware of her surroundings. I went down the list of menu options:

"OK, sweetheart, for lunch…egg salad, tuna, turkey and cheese. What do you think? How about tuna?"

She replied, "Sure, tuna sounds fine."

"Now drinks. Orange juice, apple juice, milk, water?"

"Hmm…water," she said after contemplating for a second.

"Got it. Now for dessert—a banana, cherry Jell-O, or pound cake?"

She looked at me quizzically. "Honey…"

"Yes, sweetheart?"

" I don't want to be critical, but this menu is terrible. I don't think we should come back to this restaurant again…"

Part 3
Release on the Horizon

DAY 17 — LOTS OF TESTS
May 7, 2014

Chatman e-mailed:

Greg,

Just finished reading the last e-mail from you! I'm sending you both as much voodoo, prayers, wishes, and whatever else I can conjure up. Haven't e-mailed, not wanting to take any time away from you. As soon as she is up to visitors, I'm driving up with Brooke and Kimberly but wanted to make sure it's a good time. Hang in there and please know whenever you two want to come stay on the farm in complete privacy—or with some friends (food included)—we are here.

Peace and love and tell her I'm lighting a candle each day that I'm home for her! And one for you too!

10:01 a.m.
Shar texted me:
Hi. Just spoke with Demy.
She fell asleep last night within five minutes.
CT scan and EEG going on this a.m.
Demy has seen her for a couple of minutes in between.

I replied:
Did you talk to nurses yet?
They say today's scan is routine
but just want to see if vasospasm numbers are down.
They have not called me, so assuming it's OK.
I can call if you haven't.

Shar texted:
I have not talked to nurse yet,
just Demy, who said they are busy.

I replied:
Thanks.
Let me know when you do.

Kelly e-mailed:
Hi Greg,

We met once, years ago, on a boat at a Bob Schneider concert.

Holly is one of the best people I've ever known—in terms of being a joy to know—but even more from the perspective of being so strong and so giving.

I met her when I was fifteen years old and walked into her honors English class. I went through the first twenty-four years of my life with a raging, undiagnosed case of attention deficit hyperactivity disorder, and so often (really, nearly always) felt like I walked around in a Pig Pen-esque cloud of not living up to my potential, of not being capable. Holly taught me things that are quantifiable and evidential about rhetoric and how to write for advanced placement exams. More importantly, she taught me that I was capable and worthy and that my instincts were good. Everyone has a teacher that turns things around and keeps them going, even if the years that follow are hard. Holly is that person for me.

Well. I say that, but I still can't diagram a sentence, so there are things that even miracle workers can't accomplish.

I met Holly again a little more than ten years later, in New York. There, she became my friend. I'll never forget the Bob Schneider shows. I'll never forget our wine-fueled, into-the-wee-hours-of-the-morning discussions about education and politics—given that we agreed on just about everything, you wouldn't think that we could expound on the topics without anyone else contributing for hours on end, but I know that the conversations saw the wrong side of 4:00 a.m. more than once.

When I told her that I was leaving New York, she demanded that we meet for a farewell drink. When we did, she presented me with a key chain—a foam flip-flop that she'd seen a vendor selling and made her think of me. The key chain has stayed in my bag at all times ever since, a reminder of how a few simple, unassuming words from one person can completely change the trajectory of your life over and over again.

She's beyond words and in my every thought.

8:14 p.m.
Shar texted me:
Day go OK?

> **I replied:**
> Yes. Can you talk around 9:30?
> Or tomorrow morning better?
> Hol says she loves you and misses you and said she is sick...
> she's trying to wrap her head 'round things
> a bit today and is kind of confused.
> She's still well though, clinically.
> Call me tomorrow.
> Looking forward to seeing you if you can come in
> and hope you're a bit better.

―⋄―

From: Payan, Gregory
Sent: Wednesday, May 7, 2014, 9:50 p.m.
Subject: Holly Wednesday Update

Exhausted update, as I slept little last night and had a really busy day with work, hospital, and visits to rehab facilities. I hope to go to bed tonight with a bit more peace than last eve, however. I got to speak with one of Holly's doctors at length when I arrived tonight. Yesterday's vasospasm numbers were not insignificant and could actually be viewed as somewhat alarming. They were high. As they said they would do, they gave her medication to improve her blood flow, and her numbers today, after a multitude of

tests this a.m., were significantly better. If they continue to trend downward, we may have cleared a big hurdle.

I asked how rare this was so many days out, and the doctor said that while they usually mark time from the first rupture (in Holly's case, on a Monday), she had a rerupture during the craniotomy (three days after the initial bleed), and that certainly can affect the timeline—although, as they say, they just never know, as it's still within the standard deviation and there are no hard, fast rules.

Anyhow, I think if we have a few more days of good numbers, we can get Holly into a rehab facility early to midweek, where I am confident we will see significant progress with her strength and her appetite and all-around, general well-being. I saw a rehab facility today that I really liked, so although I have to provide three facility names by New York State regulation, I hope to try to pull whatever strings are necessary to get her into my first choice. Need to visit two more on Friday, but I have a definite front-runner, where she will receive excellent care and treatment.

Holly was erratic for much of the day, sleeping a lot and drowsy as she underwent a multitude of tests in the morning. Afternoon was similar, although she had perked up by evening when I arrived. I had to bribe her into trying to sleep by letting her know that it would speed her departure. The only things that matter to her currently are leaving and taking a bath. Nothing else in the world holds any meaning to her. If you spend any appreciable amount of time with her, conversation will go in that direction. "Holly, if you get some rest, maybe we can leave and take a bath soon." Only then will she attempt to rest a bit.

It was a day with a lot of optimism. Unfortunately, the catheter had to go back in, and they also had to reopen the drain in her skull to assist in battling the vasospasms. The fact that she had gone three days with it clamped with no pressure buildup was great though. The doctor said that once the vasospasm window has closed, they should be able to remove it quickly, since her body has shown that it can reabsorb cerebrospinal fluid on its own.

In the end, it was a good day. This being a sixteen-day roller coaster, who knows what tomorrow will bring, but it does seem we are trending the right way if today's conversation with the doctor was a good indicator.

Good night, all.

Catherine e-mailed:
Greg,

Your exhaustion must be getting deep. I am glad Karen and Christy have been able to offer a bit of relief in their visits.

I am free much of this coming Tuesday, in case that might be a possible time for me to come and stay with Holly. I realize you have no idea what will be happening just then; she may be in transition to a rehab facility. (Hope it is the one you favor.)

I replied to Catherine:
Catherine,

Thank you so much for the offer, but as you thought, at that point we will be getting close to her release date, I believe, so a lot may be in flux. I think once she is transferred, the daily updates will stop. After two or three days to adjust, I am really optimistic that Holly will be able to plan her own social calendar. She will be so happy to see you and everyone else. All of the rehab facilities I have been considering have extremely liberal visitation, and as of now, I am hoping she will get into Rusk, which is affiliated with New York University and on East Seventeenth Street.

More to follow, but it appears to be the homestretch, and I can push through for a few more days. Thanks so much for the offer. Holly will surely take you up on it soon and will tell you herself when she'd love to see you.

Catherine responded:
Greg, yes, I will look forward to that slightly later moment, then, when Holly can make her own plans! In case it is simply too much and too distant now, I hope then to convey to her that the coveted award for best dissertation that she received Wed eve was almost certainly coming to her (as one of only three PhDs of the twelve-month period to have been awarded "with distinction") quite independently of aneurysm.

May force be with you.

―⸺―

I was still lost. Searching for peace. Trying to acknowledge she was going to live but unable to know what changes life had in store for us. What health issues could potentially linger on some level? Professionally and emotionally, was Holly really going to be OK? If she wasn't going to be OK in those ways, what would our new life be like? We would absolutely remain together, but would the true happiness we'd had become forever elusive? Was our charmed life going to come crashing down?

DAY 18 — SOME IMPROVEMENT

May 8, 2014

Kelsi e-mailed:

Holly,

Sometimes when I'm driving, I think of you reading "Burying an Animal on the Way to New York" in a silent classroom to a bunch of fifteen-year-olds. I hear your voice, soft and strong and stretching in that special cadence of poetry. And maybe it's silly, but when I drive over roadkill, I try not to flinch. I try to believe that I'm "being shown the secret of life" as you taught me. In the tenth grade, I didn't know that poetry was allowed to be this way. Later that day or semester, you read "I Go Back to May 1937," and again the world opened up a little more. When I think of you, these are the moments that flash the brightest. We read *A Separate Peace* and *All Quiet on the Western Front*, too. And neither are exactly uplifting in any traditional sense. The poetry you chose wasn't flowery either, but it felt real. You were the first adult I met who I felt was giving me an honest representation of the world. Yes, it's shitty sometimes. Yes, there are dead animals on the way to New York, but if you "slow down with your radio off and your window open" you can hear the twittering of their spirits as you go by. I remember you teaching about juxtapositions in *All Quiet*, and you told us that this was how the world was. It's incredibly difficult being a teenager, and I felt like most of the adults with whom I came into contact were lying most of the time. Everything they represented existed in a shallow band of emotion. Nothing was ever too terrible, but nothing was ever too wonderful either. You admitted the truth—that the world is heartbreaking sometimes but also shockingly beautiful. And to truly open up to the good, you had to also recognize the bad. I don't know how you phrased this, and maybe it was just a slow impression I got over the course of the year, but I needed it. I'd seen some of the horribleness, and the validation alone was like getting tossed a rope. But then you also said that the world was beautiful and people were so amazing. I know I've told you this before, but I remember doubting your faith in people, and I remember thinking that there's no way you could love everyone as much as you said you did. But you really seemed to. And if you were honest about the bad points in the world, then maybe you were being honest about how miraculous everything was, too.

I almost didn't send this because we weren't very close. Erin mentions you often, and I see you pop up on my newsfeed now and then, but even when I was at Arlington High School, which was ten years ago now, I didn't know you well. But the more I thought about that, the more it felt important that I send this along to Greg. I've sent a couple messages over the years, but I don't know if they ever properly conveyed how important you were in my life. You introduced me to a new kind of poetry, which would have been enough on its own. But you also told the truth, and you gave me real, honest hope at a time when I desperately needed it. It wasn't the flowery, stitched-on-a-pillow platitudes I'd been given for most of my life. It was something I could hold on to. That made all the difference in the world for me. And I'm just one person from one class ten years ago. There must be thousands of us who have been shown the way and given hope and comforted and educated. It's overwhelming when you start to think about the scope of what one person can do.

I am so, so grateful for you, Holly, and I hope you know how important you are.

From: **Payan, Gregory**
Sent: **Thursday, May 8, 2014, 3:26 p.m.**
Subject: **Holly Thursday Update**

Just a quick one today, since I only have good news to share, along with a Holly-ism or two before I head off to the NFL draft for work.

So Holly has had two good days of TCD levels. The vasospasms appear stable, and there is a collective sigh of a relief among family, friends, and hospital staff. Holly is in a bit of pain today but nothing too terrible.

She also earned herself one-to-one guard/nurse detail overnight because she's been so...spirited. Think of a security guard watching over you so you don't touch what you're not supposed to. As the night wore on, I think she exhausted her nurse by constantly trying to get up or touch one of the numerous wires and cords attached to her body.

I asked her this morning, "What did you do?" after I was briefed about her bad behavior.

She said, "I don't know."

I said, "Really? There's a rumor going around here that, at five in the morning, you gathered up half a dozen patients and lit torches and stormed the nurses' desk, demanding to be let out so you could have a bath."

She smiled and said, "You know me too well."

At one point, as I sat next to her holding her hand this morn while I was reading, I heard her nurse yell, "Holly! Don't touch that." She was touching her drain with her other hand, a definite no-no.

Holly turned to the nurse and said, "Nancy, I'm not a bad person. I'm really a good person who likes to follow rules, but I just don't think we've properly established what those rules are yet. Now I should let you know that once you tell me what the line is, I'm going to go right up to that line, because that's the type of personality I have, but I promise not to cross it. So can you tell me what the rules are?"

The nurse looked at me like Holly was clinically insane.

I just smiled and said, "You want me to answer that?"

Holly also managed to confuse one of her doctors when, to amuse herself, she began replying to his questions in Spanish. I had to tell him what she was doing so he would not be alarmed. Same doctor, different question. He asked to see three fingers. Holly lifted one hand and flipped one bird. Then she flipped the other on her other hand and then her pointer finger. "That's three, right?" she said.

At least she's still a bit feisty after seventeen days of lying in a bed.

I am starting to feel a bit better. It's been a good last two days. I think we're making some good steps toward getting out of the ICU and into a rehab facility. She's skinny and worn-out and just can't grasp the hospital concept, but she's still doing well.

Cheers.

Elisa e-mailed:
Greg,

Thanks for this update…wishing that each day brings you closer to the end of this hospital time…Great to hear that Holly is staying spirited and keeping those doctors on their toes! Go, Holly, go!

Whatever it takes…know that your cousins are praying hard and keeping you in thoughts!

She's hilarious! And, in my opinion…*improving*!

Erin e-mailed:
Hi Greg and Sharley,

I loved your update today, because the stories of Holly testing every limit and her unique method of counting to three made me laugh! I can't even begin to express how relieved and thrilled I am to hear of her continuing progress. I can also only imagine how utterly exhausting and stressful this has been for both of you, who are there with her and trying to keep her calm while not going crazy yourselves. I don't know either of you well, although I feel like I know you because of being friends with Holly for so long and hearing her talk about both of you, but I wanted to thank you for taking such good care of her. As you know, being a caregiver is draining in every possible way, because sometimes all you want is someone to take care of you and to shoulder the responsibility for a while! So while I'm praying and sending healing thoughts to Holly every day many times, I'm also thinking of both of you and sending prayers and strength your way as well. Thank you both so much for all you're doing and for loving Holly so much—she's one of the most amazing people I know, and I'm grateful that you're taking such good care of her.

Holly (the other one and Holly's good friend) and I have talked for years about me coming to New York to visit, and I've already decided that after all this, that trip is going to happen ASAP after Holly's well and home and ready for visitors! So when I do come up there from Texas, one of the things on my to-do list is to thank you both in person for seeing her through this.

I'll be sending some socks and a card soon, as well as a photo or two of Holly and me in our Arlington High School teaching days together and of her officiating at my wedding. Oh, and Greg, everyone in the book club that Holly was also a member of while here in Texas loves your e-mails and your writing and thinks you and Holly need to write a book about all this, since you already have the rough draft in those e-mails. So please add that to your future to-do list for some summer when you and Holly are on the beach in an exotic locale with writing inspiration all around you. ;)

Tanya e-mailed:
Dear Greg,

Thank you for this. I'm glad to hear that Holly is growing restless and pulling at things and questioning. All of this signals a reawakening of her spirit and mind. I'm also glad that you're feeling more relieved as the numbers get better and test results more affirming of her recovery. Advocating for the "right" rehab facility is critical—I've had to do this, and while you might encounter some pushback, it's completely worth the energy spent in the debate. Please continue to let us know how we might best support you, Holly, and your families in the days to come from here at Drew. Once you all have arrived in your rehab next-step residence, we'll definitely make a visit. Peace, blessings, and spirit.

Elizabeth e-mailed:
Dear Greg,

Thanks for the update. You may not mean to, but your words always make me smile. You really do have a gift for this kind of storytelling (in this case, "situationtelling"). I am glad that things are stabilizing and that you seem to be feeling better yourself. I can only imagine how much Holly wants a bath!

Keep the updates coming. I know you're doing it to inform everyone about everything, but it probably is a cathartic daily experience for you too, like a journal. So keep up the good work, my friend! :)

Demy e-mailed:
Hi Greg and Sharley,

This is wonderful news. I do like what I hear about a spirited Holly—especially after they tired her out with all the tests yesterday. I wanted to share with you that when we were picking her food from the menu yesterday at the hospital, Holly and I had a lively exchange. She did liven up, thinking about food, which was encouraging, but at some point, she told me, "Maybe I shouldn't have that. I should probably watch how many carbs I am having, you know?" And I had to catch myself before telling her not to worry about her weight (because, as you note, Greg, she has lost so much weight), but I told her that if it sounded good to her, she should have it. It made me smile that she was animated about food—even though it was hospital food. She then also mentioned other foods that sounded good—that were not on the menu—like chocolate!

The emotional and physical toll life takes on caregivers is frightening. Sharley's strength lifted me in the early days after Holly's aneurysm burst. In the face of what we were dealing with, I was humbled by how brave and positive she was, but after the first two weeks, she crashed. Sharley had a marriage and a young child to deal with almost 200 miles away that I did not and emotionally the first two weeks had taken their toll. I managed to push through not out of strength but out of necessity. I was there every hour I could be, simply because not being there would have been harder for me.

Statistics on survivors of a brain bleed and their caregivers are grim, not just in the immediate days and weeks, but also for those involved in long-term caregiving. Up to 25 percent of survivors need full-time assistance with basic activities, such as preparing a meal or getting out of bed. Outside of those, 60 percent who are not physically disabled suffer fatigue, memory, or cognitive impairments. Those issues make it hard for them to return to work or arrange their daily lives, and often they require the assistance of a loved one or other paid help.

Some estimates find that up to 70 percent of caregivers can show some signs of depression. They can suffer from lack of sleep, poor diet, and a host of other issues, including higher rates of smoking and alcohol use. One study on caregivers showed that more than one-third used alcohol as a coping mechanism.

I hoped Holly continued to improve. I hoped I would find some peace in her slow improvement. I hoped that, once she recovered fully, she wouldn't need a caregiver, and I never would be one. For these many things I hoped—and often even prayed—in the quiet hours while trying to sleep.

The grief, exhaustion, and emotional strain of sitting vigil at a hospital leaves you with pain that just consumes your body. Samuel Beckett's novel The Unnamable finishes with the following lines:

> You must go on.
> I can't go on.
> I'll go on.

It resonates as a conversation I could have had with myself. There wasn't another option.

DAY 19—IPAD THEFT
May 9, 2014

HOLLY WAS DOING BETTER. THE previous day, she'd actually walked a loop around the ICU, dragging her IV drips and the monitors that hung on a stand by her side. I was not there, but my mother was. My mother called me sobbing when it ended, saying Holly had looked so fierce and so determined and so happy to be out of her bed and walking for all of about three minutes as she shuffled around the ICU. Her hair was matted from hours upon hours of having a sleeve attached to her head and globs of conducting gel in her hair as they monitored her brain activity. As she shuffled forward with a half-open hospital gown, Holly's butt likely hung out as everyone's does in the hospital, but she was moving, one foot after the other. My mom said she had a smile on her face like a proud soldier, refusing to fail. Although I was not there, my brain has seared this image into my memory, and I can still see it clearly to this day.

Though still in a lot of pain, Holly was also trying to interact with the world outside of her room. She tried to avoid TV, which was her custom, and was trying to read the New York Times and assorted magazines. Reading was not an issue, but being able to focus and recall what she was reading certainly was. She had gotten to the point where she was asking me, her nurses, and her doctors daily for her computer, despite being informed that her laptop was not allowed in the ICU room. Her focus then shifted to my iPad and getting ahold of that. She begged and pleaded for days, and eventually I relented. I gave her the iPad as I went to get a coffee with the understanding that she would not e-mail anyone or post anything on Facebook. Or so I had hoped...

John e-mailed:
Dear Greg,

I just got a brief message from Holly on Facebook, so I know that her recovery proceeds apace. If you are still sending out update messages, please include me on your list. Catherine had been forwarding the messages until recently. But I want to continue to hear updates *if* you are still sending them. I don't want to tax Holly. I just want to keep inspiring her. I mean to have her publish her book in my series!

I replied to John:
Shall do. I have told her not to post anything or write notes to anyone while on Facebook, but I guess she doesn't listen. She's not getting my iPad again.

John responded:
She did not post. She just quickly responded to a message I sent. She is listening!

Crap! I didn't mean to get Holly in trouble. Go easy on her, Greg! :-)

Lauren e-mailed:
Hello Greg,

I was one of Holly's students a little over ten years ago. Starting in tenth grade, I had many friends who were in her pre-AP sophomore English class. I was a bit of a slacker in high school, so I didn't push myself as hard as I probably should have and didn't take that class. But one period, I had a class across the hall while a few of my friends were in her class, and when class was over, I would wait outside the door for my friends. After a while of this, Holly would invite me into her classroom, and we began to talk. That one small gesture of her inviting me in has impacted my life in many ways.

Between my junior year of high school and my sophomore year of college, I struggled a lot and was in a very dark place. But Holly helped to make those times much better. She encouraged me and rooted for me at times when I didn't think it was possible to go on. I grew up in a very conservative Mormon household, and Holly encouraged me to challenge ideas that I didn't think I could. She helped me see the world in a way I couldn't before. Without her influence in my life, I would not be the person that I am today. Looking back, high school was so miserable because I knew I was gay back then, but I didn't have the tools to think outside of my little sheltered Mormon bubble. Holly was probably one of the first liberal adults I really knew. When I did come out after high school, she was the second person I told. I credit my being brave and facing my fears to her. I couldn't have done it without her.

Over the years since high school, I've been so glad to be able to keep in touch with her from time to time. About seven years ago (I can't believe it's been that long), my family and I took a trip to New York City, and it was so great to be able to meet Holly for dinner one night and catch up. I love hearing about all of her adventures. She's still the woman I want to be when I grow up. (I may be almost twenty-nine, but I'm still a kid.) :) I think about her often, and when I do, I always hope she is having the time of her life. She certainly deserves it. I'm not very religious anymore, but there is a Bible verse that pops into my head when I think about her, which is Philippians 1:3. "I thank my God upon every remembrance of you." I am truly a better person by knowing Holly. I'm a big musical-theater geek, and "For Good" from *Wicked* says it best: "Because I knew you I have been changed for good."

Thank you, Holly, for making my life a much better place.

From: Payan, Gregory
Sent: Friday, May 9, 2014, 9:58 p.m.
Subject: Holly Friday Update

Today I tried to wrap my head around TCDs. The TCD (transcranial Doppler) levels are the amount of pressure it takes to push blood into various parts of her brain. It's an indicator of potential vasospasms and stroke, but high TCD levels usually are accompanied by clinical signs, so the staff and I are a bit befuddled.

Once again this morning, Holly's TCD numbers were up. It came as a bit of a surprise to me and her doctor. Clinically and visually, everything else is really going well. She looks like Holly and acts like Holly. Her appetite is good, though her weight and strength are still a bit down. She's eating and interacting better than at any time during her stay. Her surgeon even stopped in today for the first time in a week. His words: "She's doing spectacular." Which is why, an hour later, when she got a test and her TCD number was back up to 170, I was really quite disheartened. The doctor asked for her drain to be opened again (anecdotally, it could lower TCD levels), and she was given a bit more medicine.

Everything else is great. As the docs say, she's got a lot of "cognitive reserve." At day's end, when I cornered the docs and asked how to interpret those numbers, the best they could come up with was, "It keeps everyone on heightened awareness. Holly is doing really well."

OK. I'll take it.

Visited two more rehab hospitals today and got another good option. I think I've narrowed it down to two, both of which I'd be extremely comfortable with at this point. Depending on TCD levels, I'm hopeful that we can transfer her next week.

Holly did not insult any doctors or staff today and was generally well-behaved. I spent a lot of time with her trying to get her to understand why she was in the hospital, mostly without success. It's as if the brain has a defense mechanism that will not allow her to process it. We can have a totally lucid, intelligent conversation, followed by a discussion of her injury. Today, I even read a few nice notes to her from two former students that made her get all teary-eyed. But twenty minutes later, I asked her where she is, and the answer was New Orleans or at a teaching hospital. I ask why she's in a hospital, and she'll say she's visiting her sister-in-law or doing research for a paper. It just will not register. I can ask her about her studies or world events, and we can have brilliant conversations. Present time and awareness just will not register. It's quite amazing to observe—even more so knowing that, as the staff says, her brain will lump her entire ICU stay into one confusing dinner party she threw where a lot of strangers showed up. That's what nearly all ICU residents recall when they come back to visit months later.

Today I was talking with one of our nurses about our travels, and I relayed a conversation we had last summer on a long trip through Maine, sampling lobsters. I tried to talk about Holly's love of life and food. At one stop on our trip, a gorgeous dockside bar, we had oysters and beer.

Holly had her eyes closed as I relayed the conversation to the nurse. I said Holly had exclaimed that she thought those were the best oysters she'd ever had. I'd told her that I thought the atmosphere kind of helped, since it was a gorgeous, sunny day, and we were in the open air. Holly had replied, "These oysters would taste awesome even if I were eating them while sitting on a toilet."

The nurse laughed, and with her eyes closed, Holly said, "You're wrong. I said, 'These oysters would taste awesome if I were sitting on a toilet in Southeast Asia.'"

That's pretty good awareness of an old trip fourteen days out from major brain surgery.

She continues to do very well. She's smiling, engaged, and laughing with nurses, and aside from some mania and some body aches, I think she's OK. With today's frequent discussions about her aneurysm and why she is in the hospital, she also suckered me into letting her access her Facebook account on my iPad.

After I left to check out a few rehab places, I learned that she was messaging people, which she'd promised not to do. We had instructed her not to do so, for we had no idea what she would write, and how she might interact with friends or colleagues yet. As the day wore on, she also begged me to let her use her phone and my computer, just for ten minutes…just for five minutes… She's desperately trying to figure out what has happened since her injury, and the nurses and I are not accommodating her. While she's doing great, as we've tried to tell her, phones and computers are not allowed in the ICU.

Holly was not a happy person when I left tonight, although she appears on her way to being a healthy one, in spite of the TCD levels.

Last thing before I go. While blissfully unaware of what her life post rehab might be, I did see something notable on TV tonight. I am kind of a sports fan who watches cage fighting when it's on. During a show that I had on DVR, they did a quick bio on a fighter. He said that a prefight CT scan had shown an aneurysm a year ago. He actually got the coil procedure that they attempted on Holly before the craniotomy. The procedure was successful on the fighter, and now he's a professional fighter.

This all led me to believe that maybe the lifestyle changes after this is all over won't be so bad after all. If someone with an aneurysm can resume a violent professional-fighting career, I'm hoping the limitations on Holly will be minimal at best.

Anyhow, starting to feel a bit weary after a long day of hospitals, driving, and rehab clinics. Thanks to all for your love and prayers for Holly.

Elisabeth e-mailed:
Greg, Hang in there! She "liked" one of my photos on FB. I was surprised she was online...

I replied to Elisabeth:
Me too. She's incorrigible. I told her to just "observe," and before you know it, people are reaching out to me telling me she's messaging them and liking their photos.

Lydia e-mailed:
TCDs...oysters...toilets...sounds like a day.

As Holly continued to recover, one of the things I liked to tell her was how close I had become with her late husband's parents. Such statements would always confuse her. After having spent a lot of time over the last ten-plus years trying to keep us from talking or spending time together, she was amazed that I had finally spoken to them since her hospitalization—and also a bit concerned. As her memory was still very short-term, for her remaining days in the ICU, I made it a point to stress daily that Bill and Mary (Holly's in-laws) and I had been chatting, and they knew how she was doing. After the initial call the night before her craniotomy, I had followed up with Bill and Mary a few times and always felt better after having done so.

Holly would still forget things day to day, so it was always fun to tease her about our developing friendship. I would pretty much repeat the refrain on a daily basis, as she never could remember what I'd told her the previous day. It took a long time into her recovery for her to be able to process and commit it to her memory and a bit longer still for her to actually call them and confirm what I had been telling her.

DAY 20—HOMESTRETCH
May 10, 2014

Megan e-mailed:
Dear Holly,

I knew your dad before I knew you. I knew the shop dog at his auto-repair shop, Thor, who ate spark plugs. (Now that I type this, I realize it may have been one of my first brushes with an urban legend.) I saw your picture at the shop and played soccer against you.

And then I met you. And you were nice and funny and read really good and loved George Michael and Bon Jovi. And you had a little sister just like mine. And then you made cheerleader, and I was so jealous, because I didn't think we did those kinds of things. I could barely walk in a straight line, much less do a cartwheel. But we got through it.

You are the godparent to my Cabbage Patch dolls.

We began to drive to Dallas to hang out at the West End and the Esprit store. I drove my brother's truck once, and it wouldn't start once we were over there. Your dad drove all the way over and filled it with gas. Magic! Who knew? We listened to the *Pretty Woman* soundtrack all the way there and back, and any time one of the lesser-known songs ("Wild Women Do" or "Tangled") comes on even now, I think of you. Same with Bon Jovi.

Our diet consisted of speckled cheese, cupcakes, and "smelly feet bread" from the Red Oven. And Dr Pepper. Your dad would take us out on the boat Saturday mornings, even when we had awakened him at 2:00 a.m. to find the honey for our face masks.

Then I tried to be really cool and smoke and drive fast and hang out with super gross people, but when my mom got mad, I ran away to your house and your room that we painted peach and did a very fancy sponge texture of teal green.

I remember pausing the TV on the Bon Jovi "I'd die for you" part, where he is looking through the screen *at us*!

When you started teaching at Arlington High School, you said you felt like a kid because it was the same old teachers, and you had to get a new wardrobe because you and the students kept showing up in the same Gap shirts.

Then we drifted apart, then we came back, etc., etc., etc., then there was the summer when you lived in Fort Worth and so did I. That was funny. For a while, we drove to Austin and back together to visit friends, and we had to make large detours to go to Whataburger for the delicious ketchup.

I went to our high school reunion only because you and Keely went with me, and it wasn't so bad.

Connor now remembers you as the lady that drove a motorcycle (convertible) and let him ride in it.

This is my love letter to you. You are in my memories for the last thirty years of my life, and in thirty more years, we'll remember when you tried to kill some medical personnel so that you could sleep on your stomach and take a bath. Greg is taking good care of you, and his nightly e-mails are so highly anticipated it's almost funny. I love that you are giving the authorities some pushback. I am so sad that you are in pain and that you are frustrated. My knee-jerk reaction is come to you and fix things. And I will, when I am allowed.

I was super angry for a few weeks about unfairness and all that, but you were in Long Island, with Greg, and you got help, so I'm trying to be less angry (but just trying).

9:00 a.m.
I texted Shar:
How's it going today?

Shar replied:
Dealing with bad stomach currently.
Will be in touch.
Still planning on coming if I can.

I texted:
Holly got out of bed.
Stood up and she is now hanging out in a recliner next to her bed.

Shar replied:
That's awesome!
How does she feel?

I texted:
She's doing good. Bit of a headache.
But just chillin'.

I wrote to Holly's landlord in West Virginia:
Herb,

Just letting you know I have contacted all the utility companies and made payments. Holly is making good progress, and we hope she will be transferred to a rehab facility this week. If such is the case, she will likely continue putting her bills and life back together quickly and will be in touch with you directly in the coming weeks if she makes the progress I expect.

Thanks for everything,

Herb replied:
OK! Thanks for the wonderful update!

―⸺―

Holly's bills were another issue altogether. She had been in the ICU for three weeks and life doesn't stop just because you had a brain hemorrhage. Holly had not dealt with any of her day-to-day responsibilities and had financial responsibilities. She hadn't opened her email, regular mail or paid a bill in weeks. She had two small condos in Texas she rented to supplement her small professor salary and there were tenants with issues and rent to collect. I had to somehow try to keep Holly's life in order so that as she was slowly getting healthy again in the coming weeks she was not dealing with a nightmare of other issues that had gone unaddressed. What this required was trying to access her physical mailbox in West Virginia, as well as breaking into her email at some point, and seeing what in her life needed to be taken care of. Holly's physical mailbox was a PO Box, and could not be accessed, but I was able to forge her signature and filed a change of address form routing her mail to me. The mail in West Virginia that was not picked up, was eventually forwarded to New York where I could attempt to handle things. As I could not access her financial accounts (though I tried), I would call various companies to whom she owed money and tried to pay them through my bank account when possible. I would explain the situation to those I found through her correspondence, or who sent physical bills hoping that they would disclose the needed information without any legal documentation requiring them to do so in order for me to pay these bills. Most often, I could get things done by lying and saying I was her husband, and providing an account number, a mailing address and her birthday or social security number. Some of them understood and provided what I needed so that a bill could be paid by me. Others made me jump through hoops before acquiescing, while others still refused to disclose anything other than to the primary account holder who unfortunately was unavailable. It was a mess, as were so many other things at this point, even though health-wise, she was still making progress.

10:58 a.m.
I texted Shar:
All good here aside from pain.
They continue to disconnect stuff from her body,
and we will try to walk her again today.

If CT scan is good later, they will remove drain.
Hope you're feeling better.

Jimmy e-mailed:
Greg,

I've been trying to stay up-to-date about what's happening with Holly, and I want to assure you that you, her family, and she are in my thoughts relentlessly since I heard.

Holly was my tenth-grade English teacher, and what she may or may not know is that she was the catalyst for my pursuing my career path and the way in which I've done it. Holly linked deeply for me literature and social awareness and responsibility. *The House on Mango Street* is the turning-point text in my life. It gave me a sense that literature was about representation—of the world as it actually is and the world as it could be—and the burden of responsibility on the reader is to evaluate that representation and choose, critically, what to accept and what to reject. This ignited in me a passion for literature that has hounded me through the rest of my life. Most recently, I was so happy to reunite with Holly in a cafe in my old neighborhood in Inwood. We met for a night of trivia and to catch up and reconnect. At the time, I was ignited with my new project: I was going to Afghanistan to teach at the university there. Her support and her encouragement before were matched by her encouragement and sympathy after. She has had a profound effect on my life, and I'm deeply indebted.

8:03 p.m.
I texted Shar:
Leaving now.
My brother and his wife are here for a few.
Holly is doing great.
Smiling.
A few headaches, but best day yet.

11:46 p.m.
I texted Shar:
Holly still doing well.
Sleeping peacefully.
Hope you're good and we see you tomorrow.
Good night.

Things were improving. Holly was getting better, and it certainly seemed that we would be leaving the hospital in a few days and moving to a rehab facility. But truly, I was scared to death to leave.

She had received wonderful care at the hospital. I had grown close to the nurses and the staff and had trusted them completely for almost three weeks now. This trust was all that allowed me to sleep at night occasionally, and I knew rehab would be different. My feelings about moving on were bittersweet, even though it was a necessary step.

Leaving the ICU and going to rehab was one step closer to getting her home. And while that had been the goal from the time this all happened, bringing Holly home also meant reaching the point when all her care would be on me. I was not sure I was ready for that. I had become largely dependent on the professionals caring for her for what little peace of mind I had, and I was about to lose their caring and expertise. I was terrified. We were not yet in rehab, but would I be up to the task when we returned to our apartment? What would Holly need, and would I be able to provide it? And for how long?

DAY 21—MOTHER'S DAY

May 11, 2014

Lauren e-mailed:
Dear Holly,

I hope it's OK if I call you Holly, as the last time I addressed you it was as Mrs. Hillgardner in tenth grade. It's Lauren. You taught me creative writing in 1998. You truly made me feel like a wonderful writer that year. With your help, I had two poems published that year in the literary magazine, and you had me read one aloud to the class. It was a haiku and went something like, "The room went silent, as wonder entered, with brown eyes."

I remember after I read it, you said, "Now read one of your long ones! We need to hear one of those too!" I remember that so clearly because you made a very self-conscious girl feel like she was good at something in that moment.

I also became a teacher myself—kindergarten for eight years in Arlington. The memories of the way you taught, the way you made your students feel, were an inspiration to me. Those memories made me a better teacher to my little five-year-olds. Thank you for all you did for a teenager struggling to feel worthwhile.

From: **Payan, Gregory**
Sent: Sunday, May 11, 2014, 9:58 p.m.
Subject: **Holly Sunday Update**

First off, Happy Mother's Day to any moms who are on this distribution list.

While I will mostly accentuate the positive in what was truly a great weekend, I did kind of break down on the drive home tonight as I thought about how exceedingly cruel it is to have this happen to someone so brilliant as Holly.

As Holly becomes more lucid and aware, she engages much more. She clearly has some memory loss, and as she becomes more aware, she gets exceedingly frustrated and scared at what she cannot remember. I have tried all the metaphors possible—that her brain is compressing her entire ICU stay into one long dinner party, where the doctors and nurses are strangers, and she gets it...but then she doesn't. We can have long conversations, but then she tries to think about her bills, her sub letters, her classes, and her book, and then her brain resets, and we do it all again.

I'm sure many of you have seen the movie *50 First Dates*. I am living it, sometimes daily, sometimes hourly. I can be incredulous at what she forgets really quickly and then equally incredulous at what she remembers—insignificant details from some trip we took years ago. And then I get scared when she forgets where I live. The brain and its function become more and more fascinating to me with each passing day as I endure this journey. I can only imagine how hard it is for her. And through it all, the doctors and nurses tell me this is all so very normal.

As the days go by (three weeks tomorrow), I get more and more comfortable with how Holly's personality will remain intact. In fact, it already is. I still start each day looking forward to seeing her, and her eyes light up whenever she sees me. Her smile, eyes, and personality are unchanged, even now. I have no doubt about her intellect. She's still brilliant, if confused at times. I am really trying to embrace what all the experts say: This is normal. It will all come back.

It's still hard for me to watch though. It's harder and harder for Holly to experience. Especially this weekend. She struggled a lot from the emotional aspect this weekend. She's trying to connect the dots, and her brain will not let her. She's doing so well, but when I remind her of a conversation we had the day before or who came to see her, there is terror when she does not recall it.

In spite of all the above, Holly progressed more in the last two days than she did in the last two weeks. She was awake Sat/Sun for about ten hours each day. She was unbelievably alert and, aside from bad headaches, doing great. She had a fabulous day nurse who was on both days and reminded me of Holly, pushing limits and feeling Holly was making improvements. She was regularly asking for permission to take Holly off certain monitors and medications. Her nurse's goal from Saturday morn through Sunday eve was to see how many things she could disconnect by the end of the weekend, and she was incredibly successful in removing almost all the machines from her room. Holly got off her blood pressure meds and five other medicines. She got a major arterial line removed. Her drain was clamped. We got Holly out of bed both days. She stood and spent time in a recliner by her bed, eating lunch and laughing and talking—two hours yesterday and three today. Her catheter was removed. It was phenomenal progress. She is due for a CT scan in the morning. If it's clean, she will get her drain removed completely.

It was a great weekend from a physical/clinical perspective, no doubt about it. Even the dreaded TCD numbers were ignored, since she's doing so well clinically, and by now, they feel it's far enough out from the bleed that it does not sound the alarm anymore.

While it appears that she is out of the woods with vasospasms and TCD numbers, her heart does remain a nagging issue. It's still not where they want it to be, but her badass nurse, Lauren, with whom I spent a ton of time all weekend, says not to worry. Holly has a lot of time for it to bounce back.

Even today, a former student and some family stopped by at the same time. When Holly tried to entertain everyone, her heart raced to about 130 beats a minute, even though she was sitting in a chair. She was just excited and talking. It's a slight concern, but trusting in Lauren, it's not going to be a permanent one.

It was a good weekend. All steps toward a release late this week to a rehab facility appear to be coming together. What Holly needs now is what I was stressing when visiting all the rehab clinics. There is a psychological aspect to enduring a brain trauma for someone who makes a living with her brain. Holly is starting to question that sooner than I thought because her progress has been so remarkable. I thought this awareness would take place in her first few days in rehab, but being ahead of schedule, she's a scared woman trying to make sense of it all and trying to trust that everything will be all right when she knows that right now, it's not.

Holly is moving forward. Her beauty, personality, and intellect are still intact, but with each passing day, as she gets better and better, she gets a bit more scared. Until her brain resets after leaving the ICU and getting to a rehab clinic, she will likely struggle some more, from an emotional perspective. And for that reason, I will too.

Send along some thoughts for emotional peace, if you can, when thinking of her this eve.

Catherine e-mailed:
Greg,
Ach, it sounds like the emotional panic is increasing in precise proportion to her cognitive improvement.

As Catherine noticed, Holly was starting to feel what I was already feeling. Now that she was starting to process her injury, she was likely terrified in her moments of lucidity what her injury could mean to her life and to her career.

DAY 22—WAITING ON REHAB
May 12, 2014

Sue e-mailed:
Greg,

I don't know if it will help or not, but you might try reminding Holly that our friend Nancy had a stroke at age fifty-five, recovered, and resumed teaching at University of Texas–Arlington. Each case is different, as the docs keep telling you, but Nancy had quite a way back to fully regain her speech and mental capacity, and she made it. I see her every month at book club, and she is as sharp and funny as ever; she just turned sixty-five.

<u>12:04 p.m.</u>
Shar texted me:
I am not doing so well and am so sorry I haven't been involved.
I'm not sure I can make it down again soon.
I have been following your updates
and am so proud Hol has you on her side.

I replied:
It's OK.
When you are a bit better, let me know,
as Holly has been asking about you and your dad,
and maybe we can call you.
Feel better. Xoxo

Meghan e-mailed:
Great news, Greg!

It's just amazing that she is out of the woods and on her way to a full recovery. I know it's frustrating for her and hard for you to watch, but that is temporary. What rehab are you thinking of? Continuing to have Holly and you in my thoughts and prayers.

I replied to Meghan:
Submitted two options. Burke is first choice. New York University/Rusk is second. I don't want to go past those two.

She's doing better. There is more optimism each day, but I am super run-down. Emotionally, I am pretty beat-up right now after three weeks. Hope I can rally when she gets transferred to rehab.

Meghan responded:
And of course, please let me know if there is anything I can do.

I wish I could help you a little, Greg. You have been through hell and back. You truly are amazing!

While Sharley was no longer at the hospital daily and remained in Massachusetts, we continued to exchange texts all throughout the day as we had before.

9:09 p.m.
Shar texted me:
How'd the day go?

Greg Payan

I replied:
She's really good.
Trying to make sense of her stay but really great tonight.
Drain is out.
Doc says she's doing really well.
They gave her a beta-blocker for her heart
to see if they can jump-
start it a bit,
but she's doing great.

Shar texted:
WOW!
Drain out is awesome!
She must be excited.
As I'm sure you are too! OK abt heart.
How ru?

I replied:
Put in names for rehab clinics today.
Burke choice one. Rusk choice two.
I am OK. Tired.
Getting energy from her,
because she's so engaged.
You will be pleasantly surprised when you see her.

Shar texted:
Wow, yes!
I thought my bad energy
would be bad for her this weekend.
Didn't realize maybe she would have lifted me up.
That's awesome.

I replied:
If you want, I can call you later.
If not, I will just update you before bed.

Shar texted:
Whatever is easier for you is fine.

10:06 p.m.
I texted Shar:
Leaving now. She's sleeping peacefully.
Still a bit confused at times but so much better than last four days.
Will check in with nurse at eleven
but not expecting much to change.
You feel better too!

> **Shar replied:**
> OK. Thanks, G.

From: Payan, Gregory
Sent: Monday, May 12, 2014, 10:45 p.m.
Subject: Holly Monday Update

Just a quick Monday update. All is well in Manhasset. Holly's drain was removed. She is down to one line going into a vein. Her room, once filled with all sorts of machines, is now down to just one and a monitor that sits above her bed. She battles headaches and soreness constantly but is doing OK. I exist in constant fear that something will burst my bubble, but that is the mental state of loving someone in an ICU. It's human nature.

Doctors and nurses continue to be encouraged. She was given a beta-blocker to try to kick-start the healing of her heart today. They will monitor that and her head, now that the drain is removed, over the next forty-eight to seventy-two hours. Tentative plan is a few more tests later this week and then a transfer to rehab.

Andrea e-mailed:

Greg,

Sooo happy! Fingers crossed all goes well and she can go to rehab later this week. :) Prayers are continuing to be sent! You really love this woman, and it shows! Blessings to both of you, Greg! Even if you are not married, you already have part of the vows down...for better or for worse. Xo!

Neese e-mailed:

Greg,

Because I'm sure you're getting a barrage of e-mails, I didn't want to keep writing to you. I've been faithfully following Holly's and your progress over the past three weeks—forwarding to my sisters and Kat (until Laurie and Kat said they got on your list. Now to Christine) every day, before I even read your writing, because we've all been so concerned.

It sounds now that you're cautiously optimistic, and it makes me so happy for you that this is the case. I understand Holly's not out of the woods yet, but like you've been saying, she's intelligent and fit. Most of all, what comes through in your narrative is that Holly embodies so much of a joie de vivre that only special people on this earth are blessed with, which seems the best-case scenario for this terrible situation. I don't even know if that makes sense...but hell, none of this makes sense.

I think of you and Holly every day and say a prayer for her recovery and for your and her sister's strength. I've been trying to learn how to knit socks—almost there!

Our lives have grown apart over the years, but I've always considered you one of the friends that I could pick up the phone and start talking to again as if the time we spent apart didn't make a difference. (The running joke among my friends is that a good friend would bail you out of jail, no questions asked, even if you haven't been in touch for ten years—that's how I see us!) Please always keep that in mind. If you need a lift somewhere, an ear, a hug, a drinking buddy, an escape...whatever.

Holly *will* get better. We all know it.

Sara e-mailed:
Hi Greg,

I have not sent any messages to you since the first one I sent that first Monday, when we all were awaiting surgery. However, since then I have read these nightly e-mails as a kind of ritual, like lighting the candle of the vigil again, and continuing my constant thoughts and prayers for Holly, you, her sister, and all the medical staff involved.

I really want to thank you for bringing us all along on your journey with you, for building community to hold you and Holly in this very tumultuous time, and especially for your vulnerability and honesty. It made me feel very close to everything you were going through and kept me connected, which is what you needed and Holly needed and maybe what we all needed. Events like this make me realize what community, all the different parts (those concentric circles of care and love in our lives), is really for.

Holly and I are friends from the theology program at Drew, although I live on the West Coast now. I could be remembering this wrong, but when Holly and I were co-planning a conference at Drew, I think you and she were just exploring what your relationship was going to become. Were you good friends for a time before you were together? Whatever the details, they don't really matter, I just remember her describing, with that smile of hers, how much she loved you. I'm so glad you have each other still and can hold each other through this journey and beyond.

Emily e-mailed:
Greg,

Please tell Holly hi for me. I miss her and can't wait to talk to her when she's up for it. Tell her *Wild*, the movie, is coming out in December, and Cheryl Strayed's daughter is playing her (Cheryl) as a young girl. Thinking of her every day, and I know it's going to be a long road, but she is going to be OK. I just trust that she is! I hope you are taking care of yourself as best you can. Hang in there!

Keely e-mailed:
Greg!

I am so glad so many tubes, or lines or whatever you call them, are coming out. Down to one is so good! Thank you so much for keeping everyone updated. Holly is doing great! You are doing great! ICU will soon be history. Think the past three weeks already are history now.

I am tempted to e-mail Holly just to say hello and send my love in case she gets hold of a computer! But instead, maybe you can just tell her for me, if you think of it!

Also, please remember to put me on any calendar for any help once she is in rehab or when she's out of rehab and may need someone to stay with her. Or anything else I can do.

I replied to Keely:
Send her an e-mail. She will get it today or tomorrow.
Thanks, Keely. I'll let you know about rehab.

Keely responded:
We mostly text or talk on phone! Or I could send Facebook, but that seems more risky—her being on Facebook. If I was on Facebook after three weeks in ICU, I think I'd end up commenting on people's walls that they're stupid! Or say something like, "I know people say your child is cute but I think he's a weird-looking kid." The awful things I would post on Facebook while recovering from a brain injury.

I replied to Keely:
I will look over her shoulder and make sure she behaves if I let her go online.

May 13, 2014, 12:04 a.m.
I texted Shar:
Just checked in.

Please Stay

She's fine. Just nursing a headache.
She got Percocet and is resting peacefully.
Talk soon.

Shar replied:
Xo.

DAY 23—NEARING RELEASE
May 13, 2014

7:04 a.m.
Shar texted me:
Morning. How's everything shaking?

I replied:
Called this morn, and she had a good night.
A bit sleepy and confused this morn when she woke,
although nurse said she was getting better as day went on.
My folks are there, and she's getting another CT scan.
They are doing an early shift.
Karen is coming by in the afternoon,
and I will get there around five.

Shar texted:
OK. Thank you.
Sounds like a full day for her!

Emily e-mailed:
Hello Holly!
　Emily here, wanting to send my love and prayers to you and your loved ones!
　I think of your classes and just your spirit as a person often, and here I will share some ways you have been a huge addition to my life (and probably everybody's life that you meet…just a hunch). Yoga—your class

introduced me to it, and I continue to do yoga classes eleven years later, often thinking about my introduction to yoga, you! Spirituality vs. religion—I think this was discussed in yoga, but it was hugely important for me to discuss as a teenager and realize the difference and importance of sorting through spirituality as a Christian and someone who saw incredible aspects of other religions too. I still think about this often. Grammar—I'm still not the best at it, but I will never forget your encouragement and determination in teaching us grammar and teaching us well through the difficulties of learning it. Vegetarianism—I ended up being a vegetarian for seven years, and I'm pretty sure my sixteen-year-old year-old brain thought, "Well, Ms. Hillgardner is the coolest adult I know, and I want to be cool!" Education—I think you were in grad school at the time, and I think my mom was too. I just remember thinking about how many strong/brilliant/beautiful women I got to be around and look up to. I felt and still feel lucky about that.

Cynthia e-mailed:
Hi Greg,

So good to hear re: change of venue happening later this week. Let me know if you need any help later in the week. I'm always very happy to come out and see Holly, but I know you are starting to get a lot of people out there. If you want help or visits, I'm thrilled to come. If you want me to step back so others can visit, I can do that too. What works best for both you and Holly is what I'm most happy to do.

Dorinda e-mailed:
Greg,

So wonderful to hear. She is still in my prayers, and I'm thinking of you both all the time. Would love to see her, but I know her well-being is way more important! You have done such a wonderful job with your e-mails and keeping everyone informed. She is extremely lucky to have you by her side.

Hang in there...you will be back to normal very soon. God is good!

Michelle e-mailed:

Greg,

 Sounds very promising! Let her know, when you like, that my plan is to come and help her with the healing process. Maybe she will remember some of the success I have had with brain injuries. Looking forward to seeing you and giving you a big hug. And I would love to give you a little reset session too after all that you have been through. Xxoo

HH e-mailed:

Greg,

 Not engaging with her is hard! I just keep texting that I love her.

I replied to HH:

Did she send you a note?

HH responded:

She responded to my last worried text that I sent. (Three weeks ago before I knew anything.) She said she had an aneurysm and was recovering upstate. That it was scary. I told her I miss her and I love her and I am sending her prayers and good karma. And I blew some emoticon kisses. I just sort of avoided the topic and told her I love her.

From: Payan, Gregory
Sent: Tuesday, May 13, 2014, 11:15 p.m.
Subject: Holly Tuesday Update

Much of tonight was spent with Holly chatting and watching *Seinfeld* reruns. There were a lot of questions about what happened over the last three weeks and the obligatory requests for a bath, her phone, her computer, and a departure by the end of the day, but she was also aware of rehab. The nurse and I told her about it, and while she was inclined to ask if she could just skip it,

she kind of understood that it was in her best interest. When she thought about it, she did acknowledge that she was still a little weak and way too confused for her liking. When told that rehab would help, she kind of understood, particularly when informed there would be very few machines, if any at all, and access to a bathtub and outdoor space. Her emotional state was much better than this weekend when trying to wrap her head around three weeks in an ICU that she largely does not remember.

Considering her state when she arrived at the hospital—unresponsive and not breathing—three weeks ago today, it's truly amazing how I left her today. She was sleeping peacefully after sharing a dinner and conversation and getting a foot rub and a back scratch. It wasn't unlike the way we've spent many other nights, though obviously in a different environment.

Barring the unforeseen, a change of venue will happen later this week, I hope. At that time, I will retire from this forum. Holly will be able to update everyone herself as well as plan her social calendar. Please know she also continues to badger me for computer and phone access. Tomorrow, with a nurse's blessing, I may acquiesce. If such is the case, you may be the recipient of an e-mail or text that Holly may or may not remember. While she's lucid and intelligent, her short-term memory is very short right now, which is expected until she leaves to go to rehab. If you get something, embrace it but don't engage, although you may want to. Just smile and know she's on her way back in spite of a grade IV brain hemorrhage just three short weeks ago.

Holly looks like Holly and acts like Holly. It really is amazing to see just a few short weeks out from where she was. I am truly amazed at her resilience, but then I think about it, and knowing who I fell in love with, I wonder if I should be amazed or if I should have known this is where we'd wind up all along…

Thanks for everything, everyone.

11:49 p.m.
Shar texted me:
Hi. How's it going today?

I replied:
Spectacular.
They are putting her in for the rehab transfer tomorrow.
If a bed is available, she's leaving.

Shar texted:
Wow!

"Caregiver" could mean so many things, and I had yet to wrap my head around it. It was late in Holly's ICU stay, and she was nearing her release, but how could I conceptualize her recovery in the context of our lives? I had already been battling this question for weeks in the quiet times in the car, and in her room, and in the early morning hours when sleep was elusive. A brain injury isn't like a broken arm, a sprained ankle, or a bad cut. A broken ankle that leaves someone with a limp is visible but is something you can deal with. What is the equivalent of a limp that remains after a brain has healed incompletely? How does a brain injury that never fully heals look? How much could it potentially affect her life and mine? It wasn't inconceivable for Holly to plateau at any time in her recovery in the ICU or in rehab once there and never get fully back to where she was. Particularly, I was concerned with her short-term memory, which was still a mess.

How could I conceive that Holly would return to her a job as a professor, where her ability to think, reason, and use her brain was vital? I was riddled with fear and uncertainty. I was hurting every hour of every day, trying to imagine our life together while also trying to project strength in all my interactions with her. She was going to be getting out soon, and I had no idea what our world would be.

DAY 24—LEAVING THE ICU
May 14, 2014

When I arrived at the hospital, Holly's medical team informed me that Holly would indeed be discharged for rehab. It seemed as though everyone working that day came to her room for hugs and kisses and to wish us well. It took a while to confirm the availability of a bed at her rehab facility and to line up an ambulance for the transfer. But shockingly, amazingly, we had made it, and it appeared that Holly was going to be OK, according to everyone who stopped by her room—whatever OK may be. I almost let myself believe it too, although there was still an admittedly long way to go. With a deep breath, I left the ICU after thanking everyone and drove to Westchester County, where Holly would be spending the next few weeks. Holly would be transferred separately via an ambulance shortly after I left.

In the end, I wound up getting Holly a bed at Burke rehab facility. Although I would have been happy at Burke or NYU/Rusk for Holly's rehab, in the end, I felt that Holly would benefit more from access to the outside world and the green grass and fresh air that Burke would provide, in addition to a private room. Holly absolutely loves New York City, but the rehab stay at NYU would not have given her any access to all that she loved, and may have even reminded her of being in the hospital. It would have been totally fine if we had to do rehab there and Holly would have received great care, but Burke was not hosting many patients at the time, and were able to offer Holly a single, which I also knew would be important to her. As her single was a result of space availability, insurance would be charged same rate as if she had a roommate. With all that considered, we felt that Burke would be best for her even if not as convenient for me, and for visitors, being about 25 miles north of New York City.

5:43 p.m.
Shar texted me:
How's it going today? Any movement?

I replied:
Yep.
Already at Burke, awaiting her arrival.
She needs to come by ambulance.
I drove over.

Shar texted:
WOW! That's fantastic!

From:	**Payan, Gregory**
Sent:	**Wednesday, May 14, 2014, 8:23 p.m.**
Subject:	**Holly Wednesday Update**

Free at last from the ICU, which also means this is my last update. Twenty-four days after we entered the hospital on the day after Easter, Holly was transferred late this afternoon to Burke Rehab Hospital in White Plains, New York, where she will spend the next ten days to three weeks. Holly welcomes e-mail or texts at this time, and I think she'd really appreciate them. She has her computer and her phone, although for now, keep calls to a minimum unless you arrange a time to chat. While she's doing great, she hasn't wanted to talk too much on the phone and still has headaches. Visits would also be OK if you arrange them with her and if it's feasible with her rehab schedule. Weekends are best or weekdays after 4:30.

    She is making great progress. There are still issues to be fixed. Her heart is still weak, and she will be on medicine for some time. She also has very little short-term memory right now. Thankfully, she's taking it in stride. The nurses and doctors and I have told her repeatedly over the last week that it will all come back. The brain just needs to heal and relearn the process of memory.

She looks so good. Bright-eyed and smiling often. She has her head shaved in the back where they entered for surgery, but otherwise her hair is in two braids on either side. She has a pretty good scar of ten to twelve inches from the surgery, which will be covered up fully once her hair grows in. A bit of a long, thin bump remains where her drain was in for a few weeks, and there are a few staples at two incision points. When her hair grows back, there will be little if any physical sign of her injury. In a few months, we're hoping there will be little if any sign cognitively or emotionally as well.

As I type this, she's on her phone, and I am next to her as we watch *Modern Family* on TV. It's still a bit taxing for her to read, although when she stole my computer this morning, I noticed when I got it back that she had been reading *The Atlantic* online, so you can see where her head is. I will sleep in a recliner next to her bed for the next few days so that she settles in OK. I can't thank everyone enough for the thoughts and prayers over the last few weeks. I did not reply to as many e-mails as I should have, and for this, I am sorry. Please know I will forever be grateful for the e-mails you all sent to me and Sharley to help us through this.

Holly is doing well and on her way to what we expect will be a complete—and miraculous—recovery. For this, we can all celebrate and let her know.

Love to all.

EPILOGUE

wild heart

It's not easy to explain to those who don't see the wild in her, but every day is like being born again into the wonder of her strong heart beating and a full-throated knowing that she's here to be alive.

—Brian Andreas

Holly spent just two weeks in rehab after being released from the ICU. She credits those weeks with helping her to begin becoming herself again emotionally, although her memory of rehab is a bit sketchy, as her brain was still continuing to heal. She could read an entire book and forget it a day or two later. While at rehab, she hosted friends and family and tried to get back to living and interacting with the world.

She was out of the ICU and no longer hooked up to machines, but in many ways, lingering health issues muted the excitement of those gains. Even in the best of circumstances, a recovery from a traumatic brain injury is brutally hard—not only for the patient but also for the caregiver and friends and family. Never does the journey end upon departure from the ICU.

To begin with, Holly's time at the rehab facility was greatly complicated by back pain so severe she could barely sit up, much less participate fully in physical and occupational therapy. Her doctors at the ICU and those in consultation at the rehab facility could not determine the cause of her pain. Most of her rehab doctors concluded that the pain was psychosomatic. They reasoned that, as a scholar who'd had a traumatic brain injury, she could not come to grips with the likelihood that she had incurred permanent brain damage. The professionals felt she was in denial about possibly having lost some brain function and as a result, potentially not being able to continue her career. Their belief was that this denial was manifesting itself in back pain. Unfortunately, the back pain was crippling to Holly, and we would be dealing with it long after rehab in a very real way.

To this day, there remains no firm diagnosis for Holly's pain. For those who felt there could be a clinical reason for her pain, the hypothesis was that her bleed had been so severe that blood had traveled down her spinal canal, mixed with cerebrospinal fluid (CSF), and settled on nerve endings in her back. We were told that her body would reabsorb the blood, and the pain would go away eventually. Impatiently, we waited long past her discharge from the ICU and later from rehab, with each day compromised by the horrible pain she endured. We saw multiple specialists in an effort to find out what was wrong, and she took all sorts of medications to try to alleviate the terrible pain she was in, but little helped.

The fear that her heart could stop at any moment also complicated things during rehab. Holly had suffered heart failure during her initial brain bleed, and her ICU doctors felt her heart had not sufficiently healed. When she was discharged from the ICU, her ejection-fraction rate, the ratio of the volume of blood pumped as the heart contracts to the volume of blood the heart contains during its passive expansion phase, was still deemed extremely poor. Simply put, her heart was not pumping enough blood for her body, and the pumping of so little blood could potentially cause her heart to stop beating.

When Holly left the ICU, her doctor arranged for her to wear a defibrillator vest at rehab to monitor her heart. Holly wore the vest and its attending five-pound monitor/battery pack twenty-four hours a day, seven days a week, removing it only when she showered. The role of the vest was to detect any irregularity in her heartbeat. If it detected an irregularity or if her heart actually stopped beating, Holly would receive an electric shock. The vest would then emit an ear-piercing alarm and place an automatic 911 call. An immediate trip to the nearest hospital would ensue. At the hospital, a permanent device not unlike a pacemaker would be implanted in her heart.

During Holly's first few days at rehab, two nurses asked me if she was on a heart-transplant list after seeing her vest. Such questions were terrifying and had me questioning why there had been so much collective joy among the staff when she'd left the ICU. Had we dodged a bullet with her brain injury only to be left with a permanent heart problem?

Staffers at the rehab facility also informed me that they were unfamiliar with the defibrillator device, and due to their fear of liability issues, I would be responsible for washing the vest and ensuring the sensors were in contact with Holly's skin so it operated properly. If the vest detected a potential problem, it would emit a warning beep for thirty seconds before delivering the shock. These beeps, I would also learn, could mean simply that a sensor had shifted, and she was not at any risk, although this could still result in a shock being delivered if not reset in time. I did not trust that the warning beeps would be loud enough to wake Holly in the middle of the night—particularly in light of the strong painkillers she was taking for her back pain. For that reason, I slept in a recliner next to her bed for almost all of her fourteen nights in rehab.

After a few days of living in constant fear, I arranged a consultation with a cardiologist at the local hospital. He came to the rehab facility to examine her, and he concluded that the heart damage would reverse itself, because she was young and healthy. It would just take a bit of time. She was not a candidate for a heart transplant, and we had no reason to believe she would not resume her normal life in due time, although we would still be stuck with the vest for a while.

Still, we wondered when, exactly, she'd be deemed "healthy" again. In spite of the cardiologist's vote of confidence, the vest and all the psychological weight it carried remained. Additionally, the warning beeps that sounded many times during the night when a sensor shifted were awful to deal with. Over the next two months, I reset the device many times each night and made sure Holly was OK. As a result, rare was the night when I got more than a few hours of sleep.

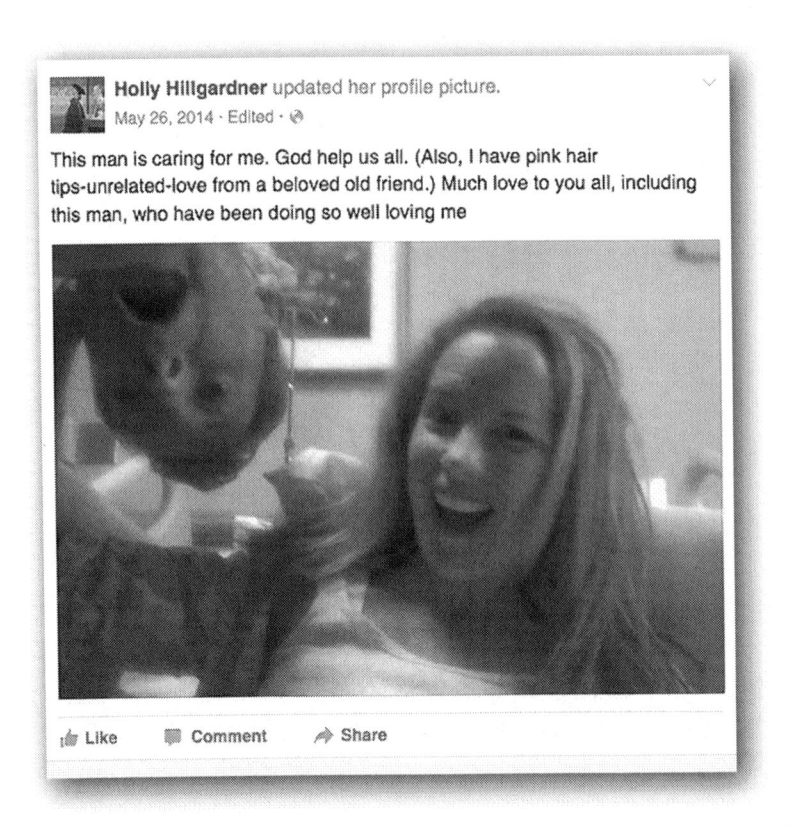

> **Holly Hillgardner** updated her profile picture.
> May 26, 2014 · Edited
>
> This man is caring for me. God help us all. (Also, I have pink hair tips-unrelated-love from a beloved old friend.) Much love to you all, including this man, who have been doing so well loving me

Holly received good care at Burke Rehabilitation Hospital, a beautiful facility with caring doctors, nurses, and therapists. Because she was still recovering, she was transported to and from therapy sessions in a wheelchair, as were the other patients in the traumatic brain injury wing. The grounds around the rehab hospital are beautiful, and we took her outside whenever we could. After being in the ICU for twenty-four days, Holly relished the sunshine and fresh air. She took some short walks between physical-therapy sessions, but she still spent a lot of time in a wheelchair and, too often, lying in her bed, as a result of her crippling back pain.

Those two weeks in rehab were a weird time. I was still recovering too. I was riddled with anxiety, and I was a physical and emotional mess after Holly's ICU stay. I desperately needed a break that I would not get. I worried about our relationship and how it might change after all that had happened. It was also difficult to comprehend fully her heart issues and the back pain that left her immobile and in tears but was seemingly not of much concern to the professionals. While her doctors at the hospital, and later the specialists, seemed to think the back pain was real and would go away, the rehab doctors thought there was a strong likelihood it was in her head. I was not sure whom to believe. Seeing Holly in crippling pain was extremely hard after what she had already endured, and she remained on large amounts of painkillers during her stay and long after.

Life at rehab consisted of three or four classes a day for Holly, mostly in physical or occupational therapy. She would attend these classes in a wheelchair which family or friends would wheel to her class. If she had a class, and nobody was available to assist her, the nurses would get her out of bed and into the wheelchair to transport her. Holly got little out of these classes though due to her back pain. Sitting up left her in excruciating pain so every class had her counting the minutes for them to be over so she could lie down again. Additionally, Holly seemingly was making greater strides just interacting with the world. Her deficits were limited to a bit of short-term memory issues, but even those were improving quickly soon after leaving the ICU. While being addressed in rehab, I truly felt any lingering memory or emotional issues were improving as she simply lived outside of a hospital environment. In rehab she had her computer and her phone. She was reading and interacting with friends and family, and just living. She was following what was going on in the world from a news perspective, and talking with all those who loved her and who previously reached out and wrote notes while she battled to survive. That, more than anything else I feel, sped her emotional and intellectual recovery along.

Visits from friends were Holly's favorite thing in rehab and everyone who stopped by came away from their visit shocked, but in a good way. I think there was a perception that despite me updating people regularly on how well Holly was doing, that something 'noticeable' would be visible when they interacted with her. It was a rational thought for those who tried grasp the concept of her having endured a grade IV brain hemorrhage just about a month earlier. After visiting though, there was little doubt among all her friends that Holly would return fully to the person she was before. The most common things expressed were how good she looked (albeit how skinny she was) and how that if they did not know what had happened, and that if the visit were taking place in a different environment, that "she's exactly the same." It was an observation that left everyone happier upon leaving than when they first arrived. This is something that sadly not too many people can feel after visiting a friend or loved one in the traumatic brain injury wing of a rehab center.

Sharley also came to visit again once Holly had been moved to the rehab facility. After what we had endured together during those first few weeks in the ICU together, it was a wonderful emotional lift to see her again, though admittedly, visits were different since we were no longer sitting vigil as we had in the ICU. While we were constantly on edge in the ICU, now, we were trying to wrap our heads around what life would be like after rehab. How would our lives and relationships with Holly be different?

After Holly had been at the rehab facility for thirteen days—which, to me, felt like very little time—I was abruptly informed that she would be released the following day. I consulted with the social worker and doctor and then took a deep breath, knowing I would be completely responsible for her care from then on.

Holly was still on many medications for her heart, for the back pain, to help her sleep, and to prevent seizures. There was a full cocktail of pills to be administered multiple times a day, and I had to figure out how to do it while also trying to work. My employer and coworkers already had been enormously good to me as I'd taken time off, and I was trying to get to work a bit more often. When she was discharged from rehab, I would rely on my parents and Holly's friends even more.

Late in Holly's ICU stay, we christened her closest friends, who regularly spent time with her in the hospital and in rehab, "brainsitters." The term added levity to a stressful situation, and we used it with the greatest of affection. Those brainsitters were critical to her recovery, and they would be called to duty again when Holly left rehab to keep her company and help her out when I needed to work.

The day we were released from rehab is one of my worst memories of this ordeal. Even though the facility was only about forty minutes from our home,

Holly barely made it. Within twenty minutes of getting into the car, she complained of back pain like nothing she'd ever experienced and begged me for stronger painkillers than what she was already taking.

Although she was hyperventilating and in tears, Holly did make it home, but she did not make it past the foyer of the apartment. She collapsed on the floor and told me to leave her there. The pain lessened a little when she was able to lie down fully. She assured me she would be OK while I ran out to fill her prescriptions—including more Percocet to reduce her agony. I brought her a blanket and a pillow, and she stayed in our hallway. Thirty minutes later, after running out to fill the prescriptions, I found her in the same exact spot. I could not help but wonder how I was going to make it through this, and how the rehab doctors deemed her able to return home.

Her back pain would never be as bad again as it was that first day, but improvement was extremely minimal in the weeks that followed. Quietly, I wondered what would happen if this pain didn't go away. It was great that she'd been deemed well enough to leave rehab, but enduring constant, undiagnosed pain that painkillers did little to relieve was no way to live.

In the weeks following rehab, we did our best to try to normalize in this new life. We visited an assortment of doctors to check on her heart and to get second, third, and fourth opinions on her back pain. I returned to work as much as I could, and a variety of friends and family came by to spend the days with Holly, keeping her company, and making sure she took all her medicines at the right times and in the right doses. After about two weeks the visitors and family tapered off. Holly, while still in a lot of pain, was fine spending the day by herself.

Through it all, we identified late August as the time when we needed her to be as close to "normal" as we could get her. We wanted to get her back into shape so she could return to West Virginia to teach in the fall, despite the odds against it. Not returning to school to teach wasn't an option for Holly. She refused to even entertain the thought.

Holly was skinny (having lost over twenty pounds) and weak, and in terrible pain, but her friends and I did our best to try to bring her joy and get her strength up. We took trips to the beach whenever possible, so she could lie in the sunshine instead of on a couch. Her brain was almost back to normal and would only get better. Her short-term memory was still not perfect, but close. Her abilities to reason and think were never an issue from the moment she left the ICU. Intellectually and emotionally, she was exceeding all expectations.

While Holly was neurologically sound and continually improving two months after rehab, back pain still compromised her life. She was unable to sit up—much less stand—for more than thirty minutes at a time. She would lie down just about anywhere. Car rides for follow-up appointments with doctors brought her to tears, regardless of how far back we pushed the seat. Often, she lay down in the back seat of the car. She would lie down in doctors' waiting areas. Everywhere we went, we brought pillows, as Holly searched for a position that did not leave her in agony.

Holly planned to teach one class in the fall semester, but her inability to stand made her think she'd be doing it from a chair. She reasoned, "If it was good enough for Socrates…" As strange and impractical as it seemed to me when she suggested it, she was quite serious in saying that she was prepared to teach her fall class from a lawn chair.

Time and time again, when we asked about Holly's back pain, doctors said, "Just give it time." Then, suddenly, an odd series of events solved the problem.

A routine follow-up CT scan on the Friday before the Fourth of July weekend (about five weeks after we left rehab) revealed that Holly was dealing with delayed hydrocephalus—a condition in which the ventricles in the brain are unable to process cerebrospinal fluid, causing dangerous swelling in the cranial cavity. We had left the hospital after the CT scan and expected a routine call later that day with normal results. The results, however, were unexpected. Her doctor told us to return to the hospital immediately, due to a significant buildup of CSF around her brain. Holly would be admitted to the hospital, monitored throughout the weekend for any changes in her condition, and would have surgery on Monday or Tuesday. The hydrocephalus diagnosis necessitated the implantation of a permanent shunt in her head to reroute the CSF from her skull through a tube down her neck into her abdomen, where her body would reabsorb it.

The concept sounded bizarre to me, but apparently, it's not an uncommon surgery, particularly for those who have suffered a severe brain hemorrhage. Normally, however, the shunt is implanted during the ICU stay, because it's clear to the neurology staff that the patient is not able to process the fluid properly after the bleed. That was not the case with Holly. They thought a shunt was not necessary during her ICU stay, but they were apparently quite wrong. The fluid buildup was deemed quite dangerous by her neurosurgeon just seven weeks after her ICU release.

At first, Holly wanted to postpone the surgery or not undergo it at all, though this truly was not an option. While we felt that she was largely asymptomatic, untreated swelling on the brain can cause balance issues, incontinence, and possibly death. As Holly sat in a hospital bed and contemplated the options she really did not have, she grilled any doctor who came by about the possible connection between hydrocephalus and back pain. If she could find any doctor who believed a shunt would relieve her back pain, she'd jump at the opportunity for another brain surgery.

Only one doctor thought the shunt might relieve her back pain, theorizing that the brain is so complex, one never knows; all others thought the back condition was unrelated. Her doctors did, however, unanimously advise her to get the shunt and get on with life. Even if they felt the shunt would not help the back pain, eventually the CSF buildup would cause serious problems. But it bothered Holly to know she would spend the rest of her life with something implanted in her skull and a tube running down her neck. In addition, shunts were extremely prone to failure, often requiring subsequent surgeries.

We were in the hospital for three days before Holly relented, agreed to the surgery, and signed the required paperwork. Incredibly, the end of her back pain exactly coincided with the implantation of a shunt that worked. (Her first one didn't.) It may have been the exact moment the blood from her bleed was reabsorbed, as many doctors theorized, or it may have been the shunt and rerouting of the CSF. We will never be sure.

This began our love-hate relationship with Holly's shunt (or shunts). Although some of her hair had been shaved for the craniotomy, the haircut required for the shunt surgery was much more severe. Holly had long, beautiful, curly hair before the shunt surgery. After it, she was bald on one side of her head, just past the center. When we went to my parents' home after the shunt surgery, it was heartbreaking to watch her look into a mirror for the first time. Half of her hair was gone, and a long row of staples held her wound together on the bald side of her skull.

She came out of the bathroom in tears. "Can we go back to the hospital?" she asked. "I think we left too soon. I'm not ready for this."

Emotionally, we were already in a dark place after enduring the ruptured aneurysm. Now she would have a device implanted in her skull forever, along with hair that would likely be impossible to style for months and would not grow back for years.

Although Holly felt broken down after this latest surgery and the way it affected her appearance, the shunt improved the quality of her life immeasurably. As soon as we were released from the hospital with a shunt that worked, the back pain was gone. Totally gone. After the initial shock of seeing herself in the mirror, Holly began to make big physical and emotional strides. A few days after her release, a friend invited her to a weekend in Fire Island. The ferry was scheduled to depart hours after her follow-up with the surgeon. She packed a bag in advance, hoping to get clearance and go straight from the hospital to the ferry. Her surgeon cleared her to go, and Holly was on the first boat out.

Soon after Fire Island, I mentioned Holly's hair situation to a friend, who recommended a wonderful stylist who, she said, could "work miracles" and made house calls. A few days later, Holly's new hairdresser, Liz, somehow cut and styled her hair so Holly could do a comb-over that covered the shaved half of her head. It made her look "normal," and it gave her a critical emotional boost.

Shunts can be fickle. To date, Holly has had four. Shunt 1 (requiring seven days in the hospital) did not work. Shunt 2 (requiring five more days in the hospital) worked, but it became infected after three months (requiring seventeen days in the hospital). Shunt 3 worked too, but it broke through the skin five months after it was put in. The doctors had not wanted to make new incisions for each shunt surgery, so they had used the same incision point for the first three. Eventually, the skin broke down, and the wound pulled apart, exposing the device. Holly made this grisly discovery in the mirror one morning after a

Please Stay

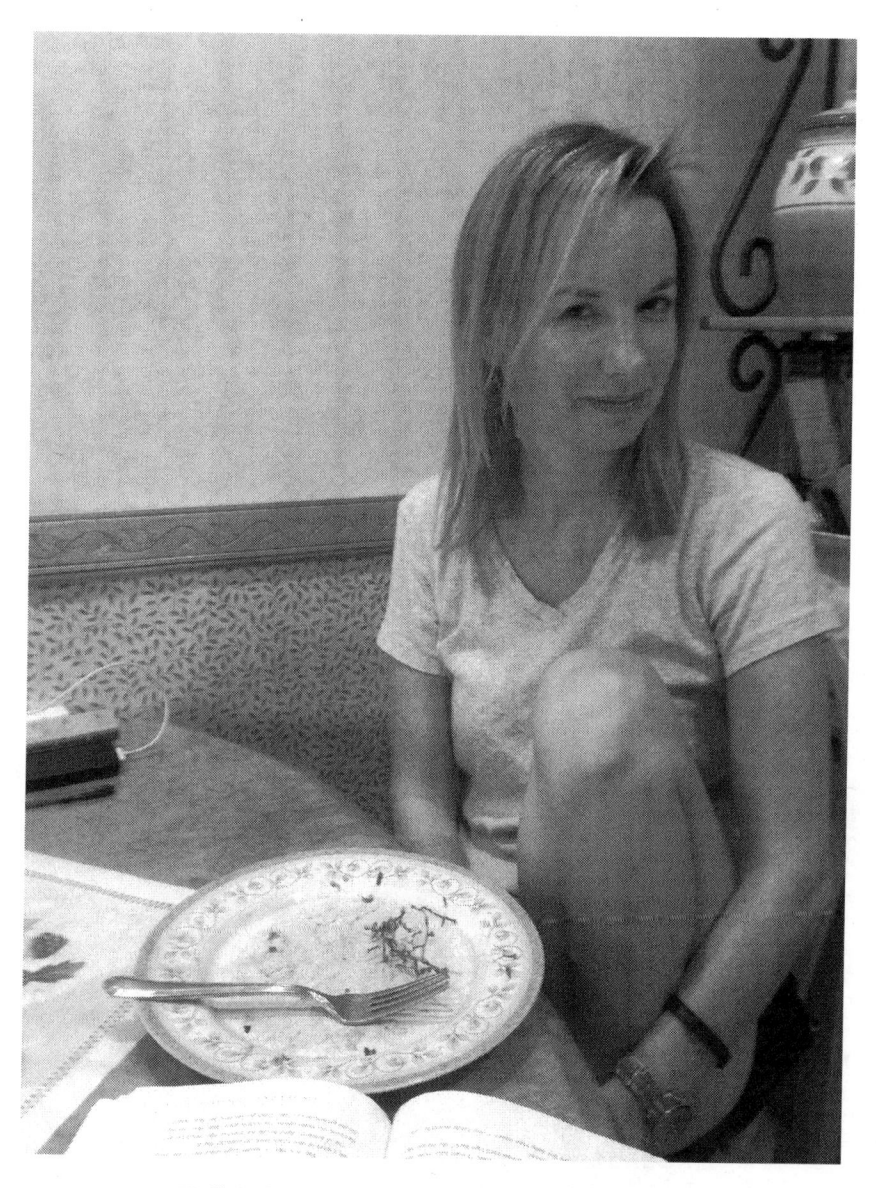

***Holly's first comb-over haircut after her shunt
surgery removed half her hair, July 2014.***

shower while in West Virginia, in the middle of the semester. After some tears of frustration and a call to her doctor, Holly realized another surgery was on the agenda. She flew back to New York the following day to be hospitalized—but not before taking in a performance of the High and Mighty Brass Band on the way home from the airport at a local NYC bar downtown. She figured she might as well enjoy every bit of her night before another hospital stay.

We are now on shunt 4, which required four more days in the hospital. This one was implanted on the other side of her head, since the skin on the original side was no longer strong enough to support a shunt in the same location. After six months, the risks for shunt infection or failure drop significantly. As I write this, we are six months in, and it is working fine. We are extremely hopeful that this will be the final shunt for some time—with luck, it will last forever. Holly has a permanent almond-shaped bump just above her temple, but it's hard to see unless you look for it beneath her hair, and we consider it a small price to pay. Besides, she has learned how to rock the headband look as her hair slowly grows back. A different surgeon handled our last two shunt surgeries, and the amount of hair shaved was appreciably less than her first two as well.

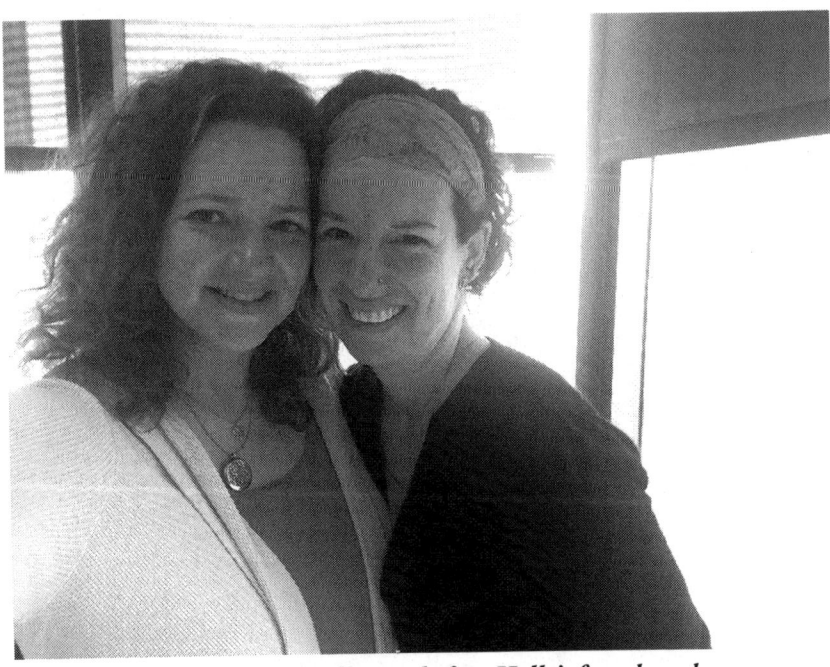

Sharley and Holly just before Holly's fourth and last shunt surgery in April 2015.

In the twelve months following her initial rupture, Holly spent almost two and a half months in a hospital bed or rehab facility. The insurance issues have been a nightmare. Her large, well-known insurance company originally informed us that she merely owed the $200 deductible, and it would pay the rest in full, because the aneurysm rupture was an emergency situation. Unfortunately, after further review of her policy, we learned that her "step-up" plan covered only her treatment "in the ER" in full. As soon as she was moved from the ER to the ICU (a few hours after her initial rupture), the main providers in the ICU and nearly all the procedures she underwent were classified as "out of network." The insurance company would reimburse only the "allowable" amount for out-of-network providers, an often arbitrary amount nowhere close to what a doctor charged for a procedure.

Rarely a week has gone by that I have not made multiple calls to insurance companies, providers, hospitals, or collection agencies. Bills that we often had no knowledge of—or worse, that we'd already paid—were routed to collection agencies due to accounting issues. As Holly was in no condition to deal with anything in the weeks and months following her bleed, I have handled it all.

She could take over now, but I have all the history, paperwork, and records of who was consulted and when, so I continue to do it. Eventually, when all the bills are taken care of, Holly plans to take me on a vacation as a thank-you. She has jokingly dubbed that trip the "Greg Appreciation Weekend." She says it will be a small price to pay for not having to deal with the administrative mess of nine surgeries, months of hospitalizations, and the dysfunction that is the American health-care system.

Two months after Holly got out of rehab, after seeing numerous cardiologists and having several electrocardiograms, her heart was finally deemed healthy again. We gratefully sent the defibrillator vest and the five-pound monitor pack back to the manufacturer. Holly was able to exercise, and we were able to sleep through the night without hearing warning beeps. After we got rid of the vest and the shunt fixed the back pain, we could truly work toward getting back to the lives we'd had before this all happened. We achieved that status pretty quickly, in spite of the frequent shunt replacements she had to endure over the following year.

Holly's first priority upon getting out of rehab was to get ready to teach the next semester. Her second was to get married. She accomplished both in the months that followed.

Four months to the day after her hemorrhage, Holly boarded a plane to West Virginia, where she teaches, as I cried a river of tears—mostly happy ones. For months I had been involved in her care on a daily basis—planning her life and administering medication. Now she was going to live by herself in her little cottage four hundred miles away during the semester, just as she had before all this happened.

It had always been our goal for Holly to resume her career, although there was no reason to believe it would ever happen. Many doctors and nurses would smile politely and nod when we would tell them she planned to teach in the fall. They were probably thinking something entirely different—perhaps that her disability payments would be approved sooner than those of most patients with ruptured aneurysms and grade IV hemorrhages.

Holly taught only one class that fall as she slowly continued to recover. But that one class had a fabulous and dedicated teacher.

Her second goal—to get married as soon as possible—surprised me. Before her aneurysm, we would sometimes think we'd be partners for life and get married on a whim if the mood struck us. Other times we were pretty sure we'd get married soon, but we didn't have any concrete plans to do so. After the aneurysm, however, it was vitally important to her that we get married immediately. As soon as she left rehab, she began broaching the subject. Within weeks, plans were underway. Holly would later say she changed her mind about marriage because I was strong when I needed to be, and she felt much more connected to me as a result of how I handled myself during her health emergency.

Holly had lived a life of loss, and I had never lost anyone that important to me. But I'd almost lost Holly that April. An unspoken bond forms between people who suffer a health crisis and the spouses or family members who endure it with them. The intensity of that bond cannot be described; it can only be felt. For many years, Holly and I had had love to spare in our relationship.

After her aneurysm ruptured, however, we had a bond that had not existed before.

A few weeks after the fall semester started, she flew back to see me. While she was in town, we took a trip to City Hall in New York City and exchanged vows in a five-minute ceremony in front of family, followed by a small party with friends. There were too many drinks, lots of dancing, and as all of her close friends and family expected, the bride was the last person to leave the dance floor.

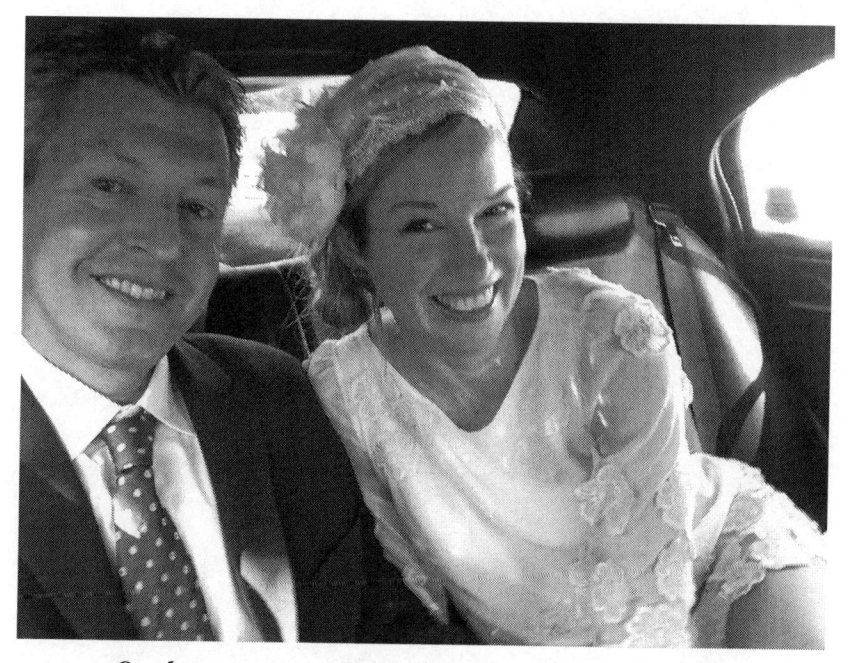

On the way to our City Hall wedding, September 2014.

Eight months after Holly was admitted to the ICU, we took a trip to Sayulita, Mexico, where she surfed for the first time since her rupture. That was yet another of her goals. I was able to give my tacit approval of the surf session that morning only after a few shots of tequila to quell my anxiety. She caught a few small waves and exited the ocean in her wetsuit with the biggest smile in all of Sayulita.

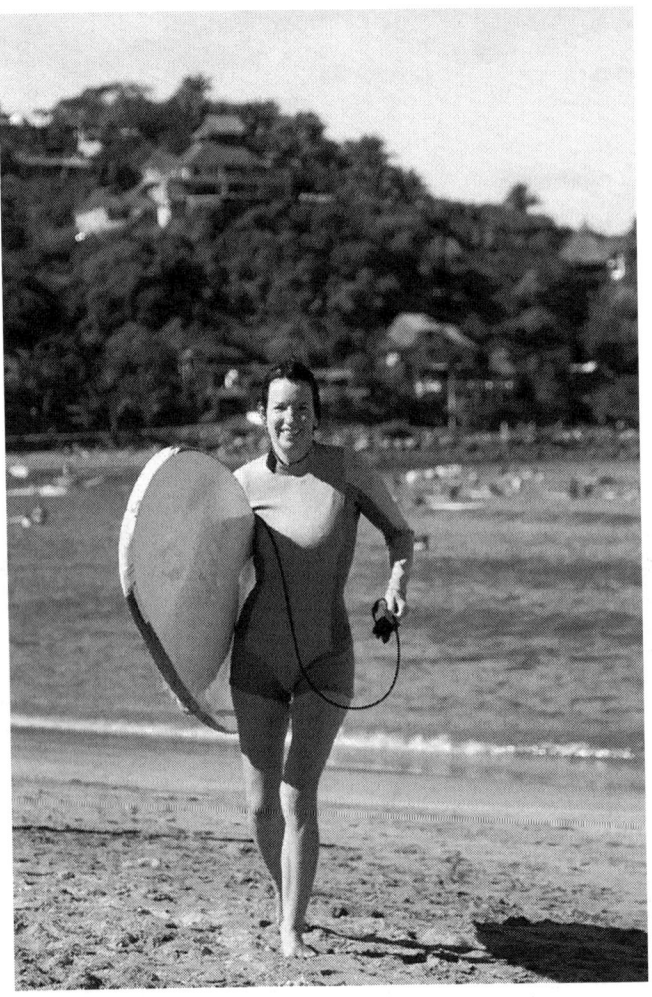

***Holly in Sayulita, Mexico, in January 2015. Her first
surf session after the aneurysm ruptured.***

    The rest of our stay was like all of our past international trips had been—it was filled with laughter; good times; and except for Holly's vicious bout of food poisoning on our last day in Sayulita, good food. Holly vomited for eight hours while I tried to breathe and tell myself this had absolutely nothing to do with her aneurysm. Two days later, she was fine, aside from a bit of fatigue.

Please Stay

The morning after her bout of food poisoning, she boarded a plane for her first time alone outside of the United States since her aneurysm ruptured. Holly's friend Cynthia and her family met her in Isla Mujeres, where Holly would vacation with friends for another week after I flew home to New York City.

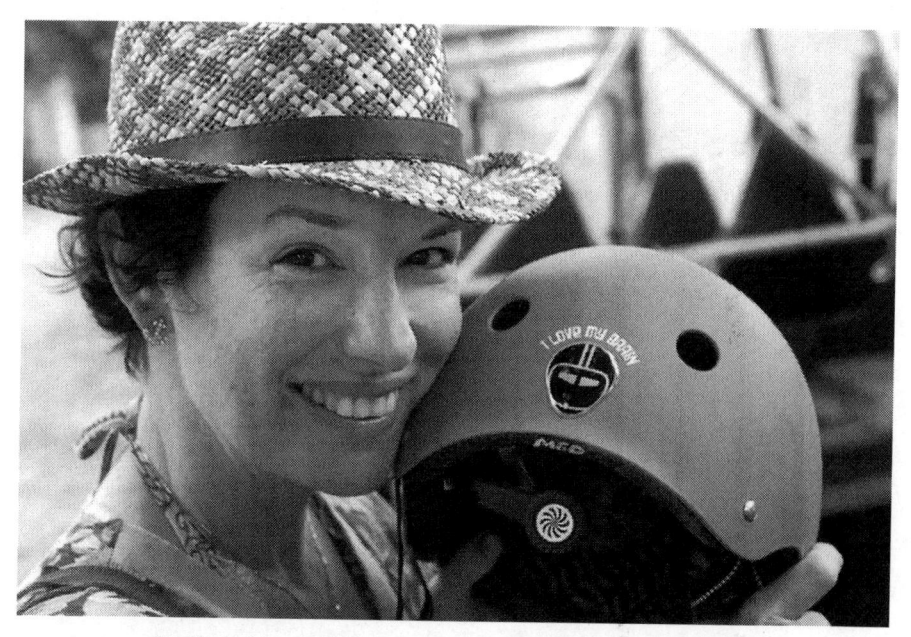

Holly holds an "I love my brain" helmet that we found on a 4x4 rental in Mexico in January 2015.

Almost two years after her rupture, we know how blessed and lucky and fortunate we are to have had some of the best doctors and nurses in the world taking care of us throughout this journey. Holly and I traveled to Italy in the summer of 2015. While I had to come back to work, Holly had more time to travel. After I returned to the United States, she chose to celebrate her forty-first birthday in Rome by herself. And at the end of her fall semester, she went back to Italy again for another ten days to finish the book based on her dissertation that she'd recently been contracted to write. She continues to live her life exactly as she did before.

> **Holly Hillgardner** added a new photo.
> July 1 · iOS
>
> This is what 41 looked like today in Rome! I am so, so, so grateful.
>
> 👍 Like   💬 Comment   ➤ Share

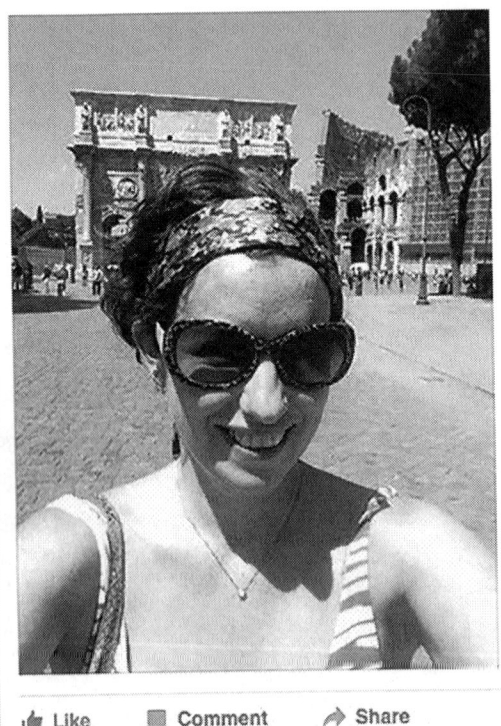

Despite the back pain, the heart problems, the shunts, and other issues, we are insanely grateful. Many brain-aneurysm victims die, and many survivors suffer incredibly for the rest of their days. Even those whose aneurysms are repaired *before* they rupture are often plagued with memory problems and headaches. Often they cannot return to work. Relationships suffer. Many get divorced and/or lose friends, as the emotional toll is so great. We are blessed to have had none of those issues. Our relationship is better, and Holly's love for her friends and family has deepened. In the months after her stays in the ICU and rehab, Holly was able to read the many cards and letters she received during those times. She described it as almost having the ability to attend her own funeral and see how much she truly meant to people.

In many ways, Holly is grateful for having endured what she did. She would even tell you that she's happier now. Most days, there is little difference in her life post aneurysm compared with her life before the crisis—other than a short haircut and the fact that she feels emotion on a deeper level. She now cries a few times a week, as opposed to a few times a year before the aneurysm. (If she listens to the *Hamilton* soundtrack, she cries a few times an hour.)

I am probably the only one who notices a few subtle differences, none of which affect our relationship even a little. Holly is a bit more grateful and a bit less anxious. Her family and closest friends would say she's exactly the same—in spite of the statistics that say she should not be.

Why was our outcome so good? I don't know. So many other patients go through exactly the same treatment, yet have vastly different results. To me, the random nature of aneurysm ruptures and outcomes after brain surgery is mind-boggling and cruel. I think we were extremely lucky to have been in a large city equipped to deal with such a complicated medical emergency and not in a rural town. I think we had one of the world's best neurosurgeons working on her, as well as an incredible staff of nurses monitoring her in the ICU. I truly believe those two elements, more than anything, dictated her outcome—although some other things surely did not hurt.

I was born and raised a Catholic and served as an altar boy in my youth, but I have drifted from my Catholic faith as I have gotten older. I've gone to church only seven or eight times in the last few years. I see God in communities and in kind gestures between people but not as an all-powerful being. While I appreciate the many positive elements of Catholicism, I have trouble embracing a religion that is not as inclusive as I believe it should be.

Even so, I took incredible comfort in knowing that so many people were praying for Holly all over the world—in churches and in communities and in the homes of family and loved ones. I want to think those prayers aided her on some level. I, too, prayed for her at the Life Rock outside the hospital and on my parents' couch during my many sleepless nights. Those prayers sustained me emotionally, even though I do not attribute her survival and recovery to divine intervention. Too many bad things happen to too many good people for me to believe Holly was arbitrarily chosen for such a good result after a serious health crisis while others who receive the same amount of prayers are not.

I am glad I prayed. I am glad so many others prayed. It provided strength that I desperately needed, and my being strong aided me in taking care of Holly during her recovery.

We touched Holly constantly in the hospital and in rehab, even when she slept, holding her hand, her toe, her leg. We massaged her to soothe her achy muscles every day. We talked to her during all her waking hours. We played spa music on eight-hour loops on an iPad when she slept, in an attempt to drown out the incessant beeping of the machines that fed her drugs and monitored her condition twenty-four hours a day. We laughed every day in spite of the gravity of her injury. We teased her (delicately) about her situation and her brain, while assuring her that eventually she'd be all right. We surrounded her with people who loved her every day through the ICU and rehab. All these things likely had some effect on her recovery—in addition to Holly herself. Holly is incredibly strong-willed. She loves life, and she is a fighter with every ounce of her being. This was evident during her hospital stay and recovery. Every limit she could push, she did.

What does our future hold? I honestly don't know. I am hopeful this shunt will be her last. I am hopeful she will stay happy and healthy. I hope she outlives me, which I made her promise to do many times while she was in the ICU (though I am sure she has no recollection of this).

Holly still teaches full-time at Bethany College in West Virginia, a school and community that were truly wonderful to us throughout her health crisis. In the winter of 2016, Oxford University Press published *Longing and Letting Go: Practices of Passionate Non-Attachment from the Hindu and Christian Traditions* by Dr. Holly Hillgardner. We are married and happy living in different states during the school year, though we spend as much time together as we can—usually every other weekend. We hope to move closer together if/when circumstances allow, but we both recognize that the life of an academic requires Holly to go where the job is. We wonder aloud to each other what people think of us, particularly because living in different states invites skepticism. But we are really, really happy.

Holly will likely have CT scans every five to seven years for the rest of her life to look for developing aneurysms. There is always the possibility of complications; however, at one recent follow-up appointment, I asked the doctor what Holly needs to do to live happily and healthily for the next fifty years.

His response was direct and to the point: "Nothing."

Holly continues to thrive, yet I still struggle. I may have been brave and made it through this ordeal, but it took a piece of me. Holly did not die, but I often feel a part of me did. In the Tony Award–winning musical *Next to Normal*, written by Brian Yorkey, the female lead, who struggles with bipolar disorder, sings a beautiful number titled "Maybe" near the end of the show. In a wonderful moment of clarity about her condition and her life, she notes, "Maybe we can't be OK. But maybe we're tough and we'll try anyway." I think of that song often these days as I struggle.

I have gotten a little better over time, but I'm not the person I want to be. My days are filled with joy, and Holly and I have wonderful lives filled with great experiences, yet there is still anxiety on my best of days. I have seen three different therapists in an effort to calm down and worry less with little success, though I don't fault the therapists. I have read numerous books about coping after experiencing trauma, but nothing has really stuck with me and given me much comfort.

It is rare for me to sleep through the night. When I wake up, I can't fall back to sleep until I hear her breathing or check to make sure her chest or back is slowly rising and falling. It's hard to hear your partner breathing in the dark hour of three in the morning, and often I lean over precariously to put my ear close to her mouth to hear air softly escaping.

If Holly is at school in West Virginia and I am in New York, I worry if I don't hear from her by ten in the morning, fearing she may have died in her sleep, even though she's notorious for sleeping late whenever possible and for forgetting to text me before her first class. I panic whenever she takes a flight, fearing she may get dehydrated or that something could go wrong at thirty thousand feet. I worry if she tells me she's tired, thinking it could be a precursor to a larger issue. If her voice sounds a bit off on the phone, I default to panic. I check the weather frequently and worry when she's outdoors and it's over eighty degrees, fearing that it's too warm for her, though she grew up in Texas and loves the heat. I constantly tell her to eat to keep her strength up. If she softly puts her head on my shoulder, I can't ever enjoy this gesture between partners, wondering if that's the side where her shunt is. Whenever she has allergies, an upset stomach, or even a hangnail, I have a visceral reaction. If she says she has a headache, I immediately get nauseated and scared, despite knowing that occasional garden-variety headaches are just a fact of life. I recently saw a bottle of Advil on her office desk, and my heart began to race, despite my realizing most professors likely have some type of headache medicine on their desk, or at least close by. My life is filled with fears, rational and irrational, though mostly the latter these days.

I like to think I am pretty strong, but I still struggle. It's not uncommon for me to have an extra drink or two to quell my constant anxiety, even though I am not a caregiver—in any sense of the word—years after Holly's rupture. The experience is not something I have fully recovered from, nor do I think I ever will. I will never be OK. I worry about Holly not only in the moment but also in the future. Is she feeling all right? How will she feel in an hour? How will she feel after a long day of teaching on Tuesday?

I have endured for some time after her rupture, and I have little confidence my anxiety will get better. I am trying to make peace with it. I believe most people would probably experience this kind of anxiety after a loved one's life-threatening event, especially someone as healthy as Holly was prior to this all happening. I try to explain to people why life is so hard, and it's really difficult for me to articulate. It's as if everyone expects me to spend every day high on life after Holly got a clean bill of health from the neurosurgeon who put her brain back together again. People want to believe that's the default, but for me, that's not the case.

I went to bed the night before Holly's aneurysm ruptured with someone happy and healthy. Within hours I almost lost her forever. Having experienced something so random and potentially tragic is something that stays with you forever. It wasn't a disease diagnosis followed by a battle. This was

Please Stay

a cosmic lightning bolt. I carry with me a daily knot of worry in my stomach that reminds me everything I thought I knew about the universe could potentially be wrong—that a world can be turned upside-down at any moment. I saw it. I lived it.

I often wonder how someone can become "right" again after a loved one almost dies in his arms. I haven't figured it out. I can pretend all I want as we travel the world and live our lives fully, but the fear that something can go wrong—horribly wrong—is always there. I had to say goodbye to Holly before an ambulance ride and before her two major brain surgeries, not knowing if I'd see her alive again—and if I did, whether she'd be compromised intellectually or emotionally. For the majority of her stay in the ICU, I left every evening not knowing if I would get a call in the middle of the night telling me the worst of news. The experience has taken an incredible toll on me.

Perhaps I am tougher for having endured what I did, but every day, I long for April 20, 2014, and the state of mind I had before her aneurysm ruptured. I was carefree and at peace. I have incredible joy in my life each and every day with Holly, but peace is elusive. I simply appreciate things differently. My innocence has been stripped away. I want it back, but I know that's not possible.

While Holly is a religion scholar, I am far, far away from her field of study. That said, there is a Bible quote that often reminds me of Holly these days. The New Living Translation of Proverbs 31:25 says, "She is clothed with strength and dignity and she laughs without fear of the future."

As she was before this all happened, she is beautiful and brilliant and inspiring and doesn't worry about much. She gives me strength every day. I cannot imagine what life would be like if she shared my anxiety.

I wear two pieces of jewelry these days: my wedding ring and a bracelet with the words "Be Brave" inscribed on it. Holly bought it for me during one of her hospital stays after a complication. At one point, we had a matching pair, but Holly has long since lost hers. She loses stuff…always has. I take off both pieces of jewelry nightly and put them on again every morning, because not wearing them around the clock gives me the opportunity to put them on consciously each day. I wake up and put on my ring, thankful for my wife and the gift it is to be married to her. Then I put on my bracelet, my most cherished possession, which reminds me of what I'm supposed to be, although sometimes I find it hard after what we went through.

This is my life now, and I'm working on it being OK. While I deal daily with some anxiety and fear, I also live each day with a sincere appreciation for my wife, who is alive and healthy in spite of what she endured. To the end of our days, I will always be thankful that she stayed.

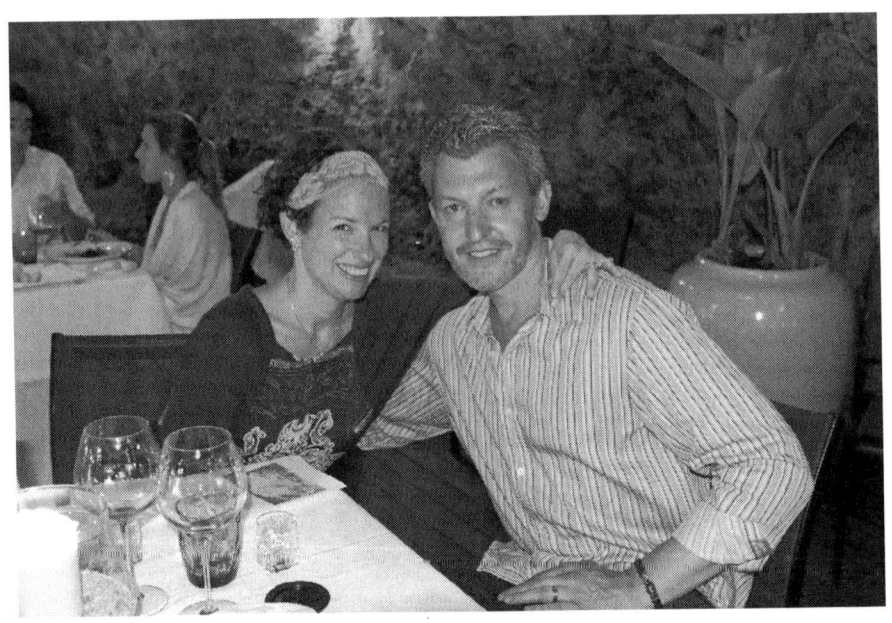

Polignano a Mare, Italy, in July 2015.

For more information about brain aneurysms, please go to:
https://www.bafound.org/

http://www.joeniekrofoundation.com

Made in the USA
Middletown, DE
08 April 2018